A Curriculum of Wellness

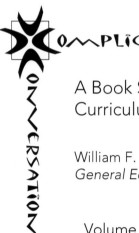

OMPLICATED

A Book Series of Curriculum Studies

William F. Pinar
General Editor

Volume 47

The Complicated Conversation series is part of the Peter Lang Education list.
Every volume is peer reviewed and meets
the highest quality standards for content and production.

PETER LANG
New York • Bern • Frankfurt • Berlin
Brussels • Vienna • Oxford • Warsaw

Michelle Kilborn

A Curriculum of Wellness

Reconceptualizing Physical Education

PETER LANG
New York • Bern • Frankfurt • Berlin
Brussels • Vienna • Oxford • Warsaw

Library of Congress Cataloging-in-Publication Data

Names: Kilborn, Michelle, author.
Title: A curriculum of wellness: reconceptualizing physical education / Michelle Kilborn.
Description: New York: Peter Lang, [2016] | Series: Complicated conversation,
ISSN 1534-2816; vol. 47 | Includes bibliographical references and index.
Identifiers: LCCN 2015035391 | ISBN 9781433129988 (hardcover: alk. paper) |
ISBN 9781433129971 (paperback: alk. paper) | ISBN 9781453917770 (e-book)
Subjects: LCSH: Physical education and training—Curricula. |
Health education—Curricula.
Classification: LCC GV363.K53 2016 | DDC 613.7—dc23
LC record available at http://lccn.loc.gov/2015035391

Bibliographic information published by **Die Deutsche Nationalbibliothek**.
Die Deutsche Nationalbibliothek lists this publication in the "Deutsche
Nationalbibliografie"; detailed bibliographic data are available
on the Internet at http://dnb.d-nb.de/.

The paper in this book meets the guidelines for permanence and durability
of the Committee on Production Guidelines for Book Longevity
of the Council of Library Resources.

TABLE OF CONTENTS

DEDICATION

TO JANICE PATRICIA KILBORN

Mom, you were always most comfortable talking with people and being out-side—playing softball, picking apples, fishing, sailing, playing in the garden, planting flowers (with or without shoes on). Your priorities were your rela-tionships with people, the land, the water, the plants, and animals. You passed on your knowledge through your hands (and your big feet), your heart, your smile, your laugh, your touch, your actions, and your words. And you continue to share your wisdom—your lessons are found in your way of being, the way you lived your life—this is your energy that flows within and around me now. If I pay attention, it is always there.

Mom, you said to me in May 2010,

> "Live each moment—live life now, Michelle."

I practice this every day and it is how this book came to be.

ACKNOWLEDGMENTS

We are all connected, and each detail of life, no matter how big or small, can contribute to a greater event. This is a moment in my life in which I am reflecting on the experiences, events, and people that played a significant role in making this book happen. It was a journey that involved many people and I want to express my heartfelt appreciation to the following individuals.

I want to first acknowledge, Kim, my co-researcher, colleague, and friend. You are truly an inspiration. I am honored to have participated in the Holistic Health class with you and your students, and grateful for the many meaningful teaching and learning moments. What I learned from you goes beyond any research inquiry. It is really beautiful to see you help children and youth learn how to smile, to breathe, to be still, and be at peace. These things are so important—they can change our world.

Thank you, William Pinar, for your kind support and belief in my work. Your scholarship and vision in curriculum theory has inspired much of my journey towards a curriculum of wellness.

Dwayne Donald, thank you for encouraging me to tell my story and, more importantly, listening. You walked with me and frequently reminded me to return to the trees, to breathe. You showed me scholarly work can be done in different ways—painting, sketching, braiding, sitting by the river, running (without a watch), or just being still. Several years ago, you offered three words to me: (i) *aokakiosiit*, (ii) *miyo-wichitowin*, and (iii) *aatsimskaasiin*. This was wise counsel that has and will continue to guide me on my journey of life.

Nancy Melnychuk, your journey to be well was not only inspiring, but a curriculum in itself that I have learned from. Your guidance, advice, feedback, kindness, and encouragement to explore physical education from different lenses is a testament to your kind and compassionate way of being.

Thank you, Terry Carson, for seeing the potential in my work and encouraging me to consider writing a book. This book would not have happened without your suggestion.

To the team at Peter Lang, thank you for your expertise and guidance through production, and for supporting my convictions to allow stories and remembrances to be expressed in their wholeness.

Finally, to my family: You have traveled on this journey with me. Mom, you made me promise to stick to the plan and pursue a career in academia—I am glad I took your advice. Dad, you are my biggest fan and my best friend. You walked every step of this path beside me with patience and love—supporting me, listening and sharing your own thoughts, helping me up when I fell, wiping my tears, celebrating my achievements, and sometimes just holding my hand with no words needed. Tracy, you are always the one behind the scenes with your love, kindness, and compassion.

INTRODUCTION

Curriculum is yearning for new meanings. It feels choked, out of breath, caught in a landscape wherein "curriculum" as master signifier is restricted to planned curriculum with all its supposed splendid instrumentalism.

— TED T. AOKI (CITED IN PINAR & IRWIN, 2005)

A wellness way of being begins with the trees of my childhood—climbing, sitting in and under, swinging from, listening to—I am connected to their natural rhythms. This is something that is part of me—all I have to do is listen, see and feel.

— MICHELLE KILBORN, 2015

A Curriculum of Wellness

While the symptoms of the declining health of young people are overtly visible, I am deeply concerned with what is not seen and how the rest of the world, particularly the education system, contributes to this state of "unwellness." My concerns began with my own experiences as a high school physical education and science/math teacher where I witnessed and participated in ways of being and teaching that work against promoting wellness. Ironically, schools are an opportune place to provide guidance for children and families to live healthfully in this world, but a key problem is that the current curriculum does not nurture a wholeness of living. It is this absence of wholeness that I wish to problematize and spark conversation within the field of (physical)[1] education toward a curriculum of wellness.

A curriculum of wellness takes into consideration the *complicated conversation* that results when we pause to breathe and explore a reconceptualized understanding of curriculum—one that weaves together past, present, and future experiences and visions about physical education, health, wellness, wisdom, curriculum, research, action, *currere*,[2] inquiry, and being. A curriculum of wellness understands curriculum as a journey of life (Grumet, 1980), an active process of turning inward to consciously understand how one lives in the world (Pinar, 1975). This is a dialectical model that mediates between individual and world (Grumet, 1988), objectivity and subjectivity, self-understanding and life history situated in society, culture, and politics (Pinar, 2012). These reconceptualist understandings of curriculum demand a wider view that brings together education and the culture large, and a commitment to fundamental change (not a simple edit of already established traditional curriculum)—this is the nature of reconceptualization: "to conceive again" (Doerr, 2004, p. 12). Reconceptualists "invite diverse perspectives that push toward newer modes of *understanding*" rather than on "efficient design for implementation institutional purposes" (Schubert, 2009, p. 136).

A curriculum of wellness takes us beyond the dualism of Western epistemology and brings into light the third space, "dwelling in the zone of between" (Aoki, cited in Pinar & Irwin, 2005, p. 161) to consider different ways of being and knowing that encourages wellness—a balance of the emotional, mental, physical, and spiritual dimensions of the self and harmony between self and others. This indwelling is where curriculum comes to life and what it means to be alive, to live *in* the world, and to *be*. Dwelling in this tensionality Aoki believes is what it means to live life, "for to be tensionless is to be dead like a limp violin string...seek appropriately attuned tension, such that the sound of the tensioned string resounds well" (p. 382). A curriculum of wellness encourages living in the tensionality between curriculum-as-plan and curriculum-as-lived; self and other; objectivity and subjectivity; body, mind, and spirit. This third space, as David Jardine from the University of Calgary explains, is a location of "ambiguity, ambivalence and uncertainty, but simultaneously, a site of generative possibilities and hope—a site challenging us to live well" (Aoki, cited in Pinar & Irwin, 2005, p. 429).

A curriculum of wellness involves an embodied approach to inquiry beyond the "epistemological limit-situation in which current curriculum research is encased" (Aoki, cited in Pinar & Irwin, 2005, p. 94), opening up new possibilities for enlightenment with a view of humanity as a "dialectical relationship between one's subjective being and one's objective world" (p. 339). This embodied approach where inquiry is lived inter-subjectively is grounded in wisdom traditions' understanding that "life has a Way to it, a Way to live that is compatible with, or co-extensive with the very manner of Life's unfolding" (Smith, 2008a, p. 2). Wisdom traditions guide us to re-examine our world from a point of view that demands consciousness, mindfulness, and connections between the mind, body and heart

Finally, a curriculum of wellness demands action and doing, simultaneously with theory—rejecting the dualistic view of theory and practice and accepting "that which sees them as twin moments of the same reality" (Aoki, cited in Pinar & Irwin, 2005, p. 120). This "doing and thinking about it" approach is relational, reciprocal, participatory, and emancipatory, where the epistemological and ontological are considered together (Sumara & Carson, 1997). This is an ethos of (action) research that when considered together with *currere*, wellness, and being, helps characterize the wisdom-guided way that is required to inquire into the experiences of what it means to be able to lead children along a path of wellness.

My own inquiry journey continues to evolve as I pay attention to the pedagogical moments in front of me, weaving in and out of the many identities that constitute who I am and becoming—physical education teacher, student, curriculum manager, teacher educator, scholar, researcher, athlete, daughter, girlfriend. I turn inward with reflexive and reflective thoughts of the many experiences throughout my years and my visions for the future. Images, feelings, emotions, people, places, ideas about the educational experiences of my students—past, present, and future—pass through my consciousness. I pause for a moment to contemplate the synthesized moment of my current location of inquiry and consider the enormity of the situation facing young people today. We seem to have adopted a philosophy and created an environment that has effectively usurped that which is there naturally for children—an intrinsic awareness of how to be whole, how to be healthy (Greene, 1973; Welwood, 1992). Again, how have I (the many I's of my identity) contributed to this current situation of ill-health for children? How has the field of physical education (and education as a whole) collectively contributed to this state? What are the tensions that we must dwell within to open the question of inquiry in a way that encourages multiple perspectives and possibilities beyond the status quo? How can reconceptualizing curriculum be a catalyst for transforming teaching and learning in (physical) education beyond the instrumentalized traditions that continue to plague our field? I believe it starts with teachers living a curriculum of wellness with their students.

Recently, I worked with a teacher named Kim to explore her high school Holistic Health Option (H2O) physical education class. She had decided to approach teaching physical education in a more wellness-focused way. My own personal and professional inquiry into wellness-oriented living and learning had led me to several theoretical and practical understandings that became an expressive aesthetic and somaesthetic weaving of *currere*, action research, existentialism, and wisdom perspectives. I believe that these concepts are the "missing pieces" in establishing a more holistic and wellness-oriented approach to physical education. These philosophical concepts point to the influence that teachers have on the lives of students and how in the very manner of their living, in their being, they can help students live their own lives of wellness.

This book is about the mutual exploration between Kim and I where we began to co-construct[3] meaning about what it means to teach a wellness curriculum. We first pondered and discussed why this was so important—from both of our experiences working with young people in schools, from reviewing the current negative health trends among children, the calls for physical education reform and the need for a new approach. We wondered what we were going to learn about physical education by inquiring into the notion of a curriculum of wellness and how this was grounded in wisdom traditions. How would we be able to describe a curriculum of wellness; or more importantly, was this even possible? What is the role of the teacher in a curriculum of wellness—how does her past and present experiences and future vision influence her way of being a physical educator and thus her way of teaching? What can we learn about teaching in this way that will help the education system become better able to guide children to be healthy and well? What role does a curriculum of wellness play in promoting health in youth? How can we inquire into wellness in a way that honors wisdom practices and promotes wellness?

The Current "Picture of Health" of Children

Most would agree that the health and wellness of children and youth is a significant concern, and while I am reluctant to add to the discourse that focuses on deficits and catastrophizes children and youths' current collective health status, there may be those who are not presently aware of the "picture of health" of our young people today. Current health research reveals many negative trends among children and youth including greater levels of physical inactivity, obesity, unhealthy eating practices, poor self-esteem, anxiety, and depression (Tremblay et al., 2010). The 2009 Canadian Health Measures Survey reported a substantial drop in fitness levels since 1981 for children age 6 to 19 years (including aerobic and musculoskeletal fitness) and a significant increase in childhood obesity and overweight (greater adiposity not greater muscularity) (Tremblay et al., 2010). Physical activity rates have declined steadily over the past 20 years (Tremblay et al., 2010) and only 7% of 5- to 11-year-olds and 4% of 12- to 17-year-olds currently meet the Canadian Physical Activity Guidelines (Active Healthy Kids, 2014). In the United States, over one-third of children and youth were overweight or obese in 2012 (Ogden, Carroll, Kit, & Flegal, 2014). According to the U.S. 2014 Report Card on Physical Activity, only 8% of youth 12 to 14 years of age were moderately active for 60 minutes per day on at least five days per week, and approximately half of American children 6 to 11 years of age exceeded the screen time guideline of two hours or less per day (Dentro et al., 2014). In England, 67% of boys and 79% of girls 4 to 15 years of age do not accumulate enough activity for optimal health benefits (Craig et al., 2009). Similarly in Australia, it is estimated that only 20% of Australian children 5 to 17 years of age meet the Australian Physical Activity Guidelines (Schranz et al., 2014).

Several researchers have also indicated that Canadian children's dietary intake and eating habits do not meet requirements for optimal growth and development (Janssen et al., 2004; Storey et al., 2009). Similarly in the United States, most youth do not meet the recommended daily amount of fruits and vegetables or whole grains (Dietary Guidelines Advisory Committee, 2010; U.S. Department of Agriculture, 2010).

In addition, many young people experience mental health issues, with approximately 5% of Canadian male youth and 12% of female youth age 12 to 19 experiencing a major depressive episode. In addition, the approximate number of 12- to 19-year-olds in Canada at risk for developing depression is 3.2 million (Canadian Mental Health Association, 2011) with the proportion of youth (grade six to ten) who report feeling depressed at least once per week ranging from 21 to 26% for boys and 24 to 38% among girls (Boyce, King & Roche, 2008). In the United States it is estimated that 13 to 20% of children experience a mental disorder in a given year (Perou et al., 2013). Overall, it is evident that chronic-disease-related risk factors among adolescents are of significant concern, as outlined by Plotnikoff et al. (2009) in their study of lifestyle behaviors (inactivity, fat intake, poor diet, smoking, overweight/obese) where over 50% of youth had two or more risk factors for chronic conditions.

Call for Physical Education Curricular Reform

Despite reiterating the importance of physical education for children's overall health outcomes, citizenship, and prevention of adult chronic conditions, physical education continues to be regarded as a low priority and receives negative feedback from students, teachers, administrators, and parents (Hardman & Marshall, 2000; Harris & Cale, 2007). Many physical education experts agree that physical and health education is what Locke (1992) describes as a "programmatic lemon" and needs careful consideration as we move into the future (Bain, 1995; Devis-Devis & Sparkes, 1999; Fernandez-Balboa, 1997; Lawson, 2009). Calls for curriculum reform stem from research suggesting that the current sport technique curricular model (Kirk, 2010) does not meet the needs of contemporary youth, as students feel a lack of connection to the curriculum and feel it has little relevance to their lives (Dyson, 2006; Gibbons, Wharf-Higgins, Gaul, & VanGyn, 1999; Humbert, 2006; MacDonald & Hunter, 2005).

There is also evidence that many physical education programs are focused on "scientific functionalism" and "display a strong preference for specific types of utilitarian knowledge" (Devis-Devis & Sparkes, 1999, p. 148) where knowledge is accepted for its extrinsic nature (i.e., promoting elite performance, discipline, conformity, academics, employment). Students have repeatedly explained their dislike for these types of physical education programs (Dyson, 2006; Humbert, 2006) and researchers have indicated that this dominant form of physical education is merely a repetition of introductory sports techniques with little progression of learning (Kirk, 1988). This approach, as Kirk (2013) explains,

> makes more enemies than friends of children…and thus fails to develop their perceived competence and motivation for physical activity, and ultimately fails to achieve the ubiquitous aspiration, common to programmes around the world, of a long-term active lifestyle. (p. 229)

While there have been many pedagogical models suggested to meet the demands of the 21st-century expectations for physical education (e.g., sport education, play practice, personal meaning/self-responsibility, health-based physical education, teaching games for understanding) (Kirk, 2013), these models are typically applied utilizing the same program structure—a multi-activity sport approach. Meztler (2005), Jewett, Bain, and Ennis (1995) and Lund and Tannehill (2005) recommend a "models-based" approach where instead of learning outcomes being achieved as a byproduct of a sport-based program, learning outcomes are achieved by aligning "subject matter and teaching strategies that aim specifically and explicitly to achieve health-related outcomes" (Kirk, 2013, p. 225).

Missing from these types of models, kits, and strategies, however, is the idea that children already have an intrinsic awareness of how to be healthy (Freire, as cited in Greene, 1971), and as long as we continue to address curriculum in a technical "ends-means" way, physical education's long-term goal of healthy active living will continue to elude our children and youth. Therefore, there is a call for a more holistic approach to physical education curriculum (Lodewyk, Lu, & Kentel, 2009; Kilborn, Lorusso & Francis, 2015) where "health becomes part of students' lives, not a set of scientific facts" (St. Leger, 2004, p. 405) and where we focus on living life *in* the world, connected to the self and each other (Smith, 2011a). It calls for a more open, humanistic, and ontological way of knowing and encourages a vision of curriculum that is based on the pedagogical ontology of subjective experiences (Carr & Kemmis, 2009).

A Wellness Approach

If the expectation is that "physical education can make a meaningful contribution to a range of urgent social issues such as health" (Kirk, 2013, p. 224), then understanding the genealogy (root meaning) of health and wellness is a good place to begin to "rethink" curriculum in physical education. *Well* (O.E. 1650) meaning "in a satisfactory manner" is the "quality or state of being healthy in body and mind, especially as the result of deliberate effort" (well, n.d.). *Health* (1550, O.E. *hælþ*) means "wholeness, a being whole, sound or well" (health, n.d.).

A wellness approach that considers body, mind, and spirit provides a perspective that is needed to embrace subjective knowledge in physical education and student health in a holistic way. Lu, Tito and Kentel (2009) believe that subjective knowledge "figure[s] into one's being, one's health and one's fitness, and a physical education that ignores this is simply incomplete" (p. 355). Rintala (1991) supports the idea of nondualistic[4] thinking of body and mind, and recognizes the positive impact it could have on physical education curricula. Bain (1995) also explains how physical education should let go of "striving and judgment" (p. 250), embrace the concept of mindfulness, and become more balanced in scientific and subjective knowledge.

The idea of a wellness-related curriculum is not entirely new and has recently been discussed in the province of Alberta in the *Framework for Kindergarten to Grade 12 Wellness Education* (Alberta Education, 2009). Within this framework, education stakeholders have defined wellness as

> a balanced state of emotional, intellectual, physical, social, and spiritual wellbeing that enables students to reach their full potential in the school community. Personal wellness occurs with commitment to lifestyle choices based on healthy attitudes and actions. (Alberta Education, 2009, p. 3)

A key component of this definition is that wellness is dependent upon taking care of the whole self—body, mind, and spirit, and the reference of a connectedness to others, to community. This type of thinking captures some of the key characteristics of wisdom traditions, a theoretical underpinning of wellness. The value of wisdom traditions is that they help us re-examine our world from a point of view that demands consciousness, mindfulness, and connections between the mind, body, and heart. They challenge us to be aware of how the smallest details of life are connected to the most significant of events (Kornfield, 2000; Smith, 2011a). A common thread among all wisdom traditions is the notion that health is intrinsic and already present within us[5] (Smith, 2011a; Kabat-Zinn, 1990), and that the source of wellness is wakeful awareness (Toelken, 1976; Welwood, 1992). This mindfulness connects the individual—body, mind, and spirit—to the collective wellbeing of society.

Rethinking Physical Education Curriculum

Shifting to a wellness approach also requires a different perspective of the notion of curriculum itself. In Greene's (1971) article "Curriculum and Consciousness," she describes how curriculum from the learner's perspective is often regarded as just an "arrangement of subjects, a structure of socially prescribed knowledge" (p. 135). She is concerned that we do not allow students to make sense of their learning according to their own life-worlds:

> Preoccupied with priorities, purposes, programs of "intended learning" and intended (or unintended) manipulation, we pay too little attention to the individual in quest

of his own future, bent on surpassing what is merely "given," on breaking through the everyday. We are still too prone to dichotomize: to think of "disciplines" or "public traditions" or "accumulated wisdom" or "common culture" as objectively existent to the knower—there to be discovered, mastered, learned. (p. 135)

In physical education, our curriculum activities often promote a lack of consciousness and awareness of the body, impacting an individual's ability to live healthfully because the source of motivation is external and imposed. Physical activity needs to be experienced and understood holistically, and existential perspectives may be one way to provoke this holistic connectivity.

There is evidence that some physical education teachers and researchers are working toward changing curriculum perspectives. For example, Gibbons and Gaul (2004) used a dialogical curriculum development process for a girls-only physical education class that actively sought input from students and included features such as emphasis on lifetime physical activities, personal physical activity goal setting, social support strategies to encourage students, and an emphasis on health-related knowledge. Halas (2002) highlights a physical education program that prioritized participation over skill ability, de-emphasized winning, offered a safe and fair environment, included students' input on the daily curriculum, and helped nurture positive and encouraging relationships between students and adult role models. Butler's (2006) work in games education challenges curriculum constructions by demonstrating inherent and intrinsic value for learners. This approach also encourages physical educators to reflect on their own value orientations to be able to consider curriculum as praxis.

Changing the way we think about curriculum is a possible solution for physical education reform, and the notion of *currere* provides an alternate perspective that could positively impact teachers' wellbeing, their way of being a teacher, and their ability to guide students to holistic health.

Curriculum as *Currere*

Currently, the taken-for-granted understanding of many physical education teachers is to regard the curriculum as a document outlining the set of learning outcomes that guide classroom activities. A reconceptualized notion of curriculum however involves understanding curriculum as "political, historical and autobiographical text" (Pinar, Reynolds, Slattery & Taubman, 2004, p. 223). Further, Pinar (2012) has argued for the reconceptualization of curriculum as *currere*—running the course of life, in which curriculum becomes active, subjective, social—a conversation about our lives and how we live them. Understanding curriculum as *currere* provides a new way of thinking about teaching physical education where we understand that our *being* cannot be separated from the world, and thus our location as human beings—temporally, spatially, and socially—must be understood as intimately connected to our embodied experiences with history and culture. In addition, this focus on curriculum as "the journey of life" (Grumet, 1980) is necessary for a holistic vision of physical education to emerge where teachers can begin to understand the subjectivities of themselves and their students. Thinking of curriculum as *currere* also opens up the possibility for discussion of how existentialist views can influence teachers' notions of teaching in the physical education setting and their understanding of teaching practice.

Teaching as a Way of Being

An existentialist perspective challenges us to be reflective, to pay "full attention to life" (Greene, 1977, p. 123), and as a theoretical framework is primarily concerned with the question of existence and what it means "to be." In educational research, the existential lens helps us distinguish between "the act of teaching from *being* a teacher" (Feldman, 2009, p. 381) and presents the ontological questions: "Who am I as a teacher? How does the way I am a teacher affect how I teach?" (Feldman, 2009, p. 381). In educational philosophy, this idea of human *becoming* is more than just about learning and experiencing the world, it includes understanding the "full situatedness of the individuals and their acknowledgements of their projects" (Feldman, 2009, p. 383). This philosophy is about a "mode of being-with-others," "relating *with* students," (Aoki, cited in Pinar & Irwin, 2005, p. 361) and "an understanding of teachers and students as embodied beings of wholeness" (p. 362).

Typically, the nature of physical education is focused on "practice" (related to *techne*) guided by preconceived activities and standards of performance. The idea of teaching as "a way of being" allows us to consider practice differently, as *phronesis*—knowledge from the practical disciplines that is dialectical in thought and action and grounded in a "moral disposition to act truly and justly" (Carr & Kemmis, 1986, p. 33). The concept of phronesis is a key philosophical perspective for physical education because it supports the need for a dialectical, reflexive process (Carr & Kemmis, 1986) that reflects the characteristic of the social setting and the humanistic nature of the physical education environment. Dunne (1993) further explains that phronesis "characterizes a person who knows how to live well (*eu zen*)" (p. 244). To guide our children and youth to live healthfully in this world, it is important for teachers to also know how to live well. This wellness way of *being* a teacher has the potential to change how we think about living curriculum in (physical) education, which is the focus of this book.

The Journey to Wellness

This book seeks to encourage a deeper discussion about teaching (guiding) our children how to be healthy, how to live well. While educators in schools and universities have recognized the importance of a healthy active-living approach in physical education, these goals have been slow to be realized in practice. For several years, many in the field of physical education have been asking why we continue to see "more of the same" (Kirk, 2010, p. 122) in our schools' physical and health education programs. Humbert (2005) expressed students' frustration that they have been bouncing the same "balls since grade three" (p. 11) and suggests, "we must respond to their changing needs and interests" (p. 11). Within the field, attention to instructional models, strategies, efficiencies, and primarily objective ways of researching and knowing are common. But students are expressing different needs that challenge us to draw our attention to individual and collective subjectivities, and to accept other ways of knowing and being.

An aspiration of this book is not only to share the ontological way of being a teacher but to guide the reader through my own journey and Kim's journey of exploration and enlightenment for meaningful ways to understand the relationships within and among self, other, and the natural world. Through a wisdom-guided inquiry process that weaves together the method of *currere*, action research, existentialism, and wisdom perspectives, Kim and I consider the question: what does it mean to teach a wellness curriculum in physical education? I will forewarn readers that the regressive, progressive, and analytical moments of the autobiographical process of *currere* may at times seem critical of our individual selves and the field of physical education but in the end this series of personal and social pedagogical encounters facilitated a difficult transition to "deeper levels of being, knowing and engagement" (Eppert & Wang, 2008, p. xviii) that may be helpful for inspiring others to negotiate subjectivity in physical education and begin to (re)envision teaching children how to take care of their whole selves—body, mind, and spirit.

By sharing Kim and my journey(s)—individually and together—to (re) (dis)cover a curriculum of wellness, I endeavor to facilitate a more *complicated conversation*[6] about physical education within the context of curriculum studies by embedding wisdom and existential perspectives, and reconceptualist curriculum theory. I acknowledge and respect the efforts of teachers and researchers in physical education who are, like myself, engaged in ongoing inquiry and discussion to present new insights that breathe life forces into the conversation, insights that have been lacking, that have affected our balance as a whole discipline. It is my hope that our stories, insights, and learning contribute to balance and harmony for ourselves, our children, and our field.

A final note about how the book is organized. The introduction provides a rationale about the need for curriculum reform in physical education and presents background information and research on the health status of children and youth, wellness, reconceptualized notions of curriculum, curriculum as *currere*, and existential perspectives of teaching. I also propose that to address the issue of curricular reform in physical education, we need to explore teachers living a curriculum of wellness with their students.

Chapter 1 explains the relationality of the theoretical perspectives in this inquiry, offers a different way to live as a researcher, and presents the notion of wisdom-guided inquiry. The chapter begins by introducing readers to Kim, the teacher who participated as a co-researcher in this inquiry into a curriculum of wellness. There is important emphasis on the nature of the co-researcher relationship and how a collaborative, reciprocal, and democratic relationship is imperative to be able to co-construct meaning. The stages of the inquiry process that involved researcher-as-participant, researcher-as-observer, and teacher-researcher are outlined and the theoretical concepts of wisdom, *currere*, and action research are connected as a mode of inquiry. The chapter concludes with a discussion about how I came to live and understand this inquiry process as being unique—a wisdom-guided way of inquiry.

Chapter 2 takes readers through my process of discovering the theoretical underpinnings for this book. Here, I share how I was introduced to Maxine Greene, one of the foremost educational philosophers of our time, as well as curriculum theorists William Pinar and Madeleine Grumet, and outline how I came to understand a reconceptualized understanding of curriculum. These were key progressive events for restoring my energy to follow my passion for wellness in physical education. I then outline how my investigation into action research helped me understand how *action research as an ethos* lends itself well to curriculum inquiry. My journey then led me to wisdom traditions and I began to see connections between all the theoretical lenses—the idea that "life has a *Way* to it, a *Way* to live that is compatible with, or co-extensive with the very manner of Life's unfolding" (Smith, 2008a, p. 2). I conclude the chapter by providing a brief background and overview of wisdom traditions.

Chapter 3 marks the beginning of my own journey through a curriculum inquiry process that involved the autobiographical method of *currere*. I highlight past events, experiences, and people, and visions for the future that were significant to my identity as a teacher, teacher educator, and researcher in physical education, and analyze them by connecting and integrating appropriate literature. This section is important because as Smith (2011b) says, "*Who* is doing the research is just as important as *what* research is being done and *how*" (p. 5). My own *currere* process is also critical to this study, as I was then able to share my experiences and further analyze my own regressive and progressive moments together with Kim.

Chapter 4 captures the essence of this new mode of curriculum inquiry by detailing the inquiry journey and realizing that within the inquiry journey is where the pedagogical moments lie. The process of *currere*, where the regressive, progressive, and analytical moments dynamically intertwine within the energy of the body, mind, spirit, and heart to constantly co-create and synthesize the present—this is a journey that I lived with a teacher to begin a conversation about how to be whole, how to guide children to live healthfully. Synthesis—make it all whole. Health (1550, O.E. *hælþ*) means "wholeness, a being whole, sound or well." Thus the story of the inquiry process is integral to how we represent the nature of teaching and living in a way that helps students to live well. This chapter highlights the key components: the *currere* process, our way of living as co-researchers, and my reflections as an observer and participant in the physical education classroom. It draws attention to how the teaching situation is filled with many different encounters and experiences that connect us to a certain historical, political, cultural, and economic condition, and how we must inquire in *a way* that allows us to respond mindfully and pedagogically (Smith, 2013).

Chapter 5 characterizes how Kim participates in a curriculum of wellness in a physical education with her students and attempts to portray *the way* a teacher is with her students to help them learn how to live well. These descriptions and stories are meant to be woven with the inquiry journey stories from Chapter 5 to offer a more (w)holistic vision on how to teach in a wisdom-guided, wellness-oriented way.

In Chapter 6 the reader is brought full circle to a location where I synthesize the pedagogical moments that have been analyzed throughout the high school semester. As co-researchers, we struggle with the notion of "answering" the research question and suggest abandoning our focus on an end-product solution and instead begin learning from the journey to allow an opportunity for a deeper understanding of the real dilemmas that are present. Four "big ideas" are offered as discussion points that when woven with the experience of the ontological, axiological, cosmological, and epistemological knowledge(s) that were expressed in previous chapters provide a basis for people to go on their own journeys to understand what it means to teach in this way.

Chapter 7 offers a personal perspective about my present location and synthetical moment of inquiry. It (re)turns the reader to the location where, when, and how I started, restart, and continue my journey, (re)connecting with a meditative sensibility that recovers the unity of body, mind, and spirit so that we are better able to live healthfully *in* the world.

· 1 ·

SETTING THE STAGE FOR WELLNESS

Tune into the process and flux of life with all its uncertainties, vicissitudes, incon-
sistencies, and ambiguities.... They reach the subjective realities, pull in the historic
and contextualize the present within the total framework of individual lives.
— PETER WOODS, 1985 (CITED IN BRITZMAN, 1991, P. 67)

I first met Kim many years ago when I was a curriculum manager for the provincial department of education. She had come to the department to advocate
for her Holistic Health Option physical education course to be recognized as
a provincial course. Ironically, due to policy restrictions and procedures, we
turned her down. But her passion and ideas made an impression and several
years later when I was pondering the notion of wellness in physical education,
her spirit and vision once again found its way to my consciousness. I immediately contacted her, and over coffee we discussed my desire to inquire into a
curriculum of wellness.

Kim was a graduate of the University of Alberta teacher education program and I was intrigued when my supervisor told me about her success as
a varsity athlete and later on a provincial club coach and varsity assistant
coach. I wondered about her story and how she came to teach a holistic health
course when she was previously focused on winning provincial championships
and appeared to be teaching in a traditional physical education setting. Did
she experience the same type of enlightenment that I did to have a vision of

a wellness approach? What significant events and experiences contributed to her shifting her approach? Or perhaps she had always taught this way? Since I was looking for an existing wellness-oriented program, I approached Kim to ask her if she would be interested in this potential research project and she agreed with enthusiasm.

Kim teaches in an urban public high school (grades 10 through 12) in Alberta, Canada. Her school is situated in a large school district that has approximately 13 senior high schools (grades 10–12), 27 junior high schools (grades 7–9), 124 elementary schools (grades K–6) and a student population of approximately 80,000 (Alberta Education, 2013). At the time of our working together, the student enrollment was approximately 1,950 and the school had 100 teaching staff members, eight of whom were physical education teachers. In the province of Alberta, only the Physical Education 10 course is required for graduation, but there are other physical education–related grade 10, 11, and 12 courses available for students to choose as electives. This physical education department offers several elective courses at all three grade levels including: Physical Education, Holistic Health Option, and Sport Performance. The school also hosts three sport academy programs: golf, hockey, and women's soccer. They have a well-developed extra-curricular athletics program with more than 17 different sports, 40 teams, and more than 1,000 student athletes.

At the time, Kim was 35 years old with 12 years of teaching experience at the high school level. She has two major teaching areas, physical education and social studies, but has since added teaching psychology and yoga. During the semester we worked together, Kim taught two Holistic Health Option classes and two social studies classes. In addition, she volunteered to assist with the senior girls' volleyball team as the teacher sponsor, organized a major basketball tournament for the region and coordinated the school staff social committee. Kim's background experience and journey to becoming a teacher of the Holistic Health Option course are an integral part how we co-constructed meaning about teaching a wellness-oriented approach.

The course we focused our inquiry on was titled Holistic Health Option, which she aptly abbreviated to "H2O." It's an appropriate metaphor when you consider that water is such an essential element to health, wholeness, balance, and harmony. As the inquiry was my idea, I obviously already had a question in mind; however, in my initial conversation with Kim I knew I had to be open to modifying my plan to ensure that her values were reflected in the inquiry process (Winter, 2003). In other words, Kim had to feel that the inquiry was something she was comfortable with and felt would be beneficial for her interests and needs. During our first discussion she was very clear about what she wanted. First, she wanted to be able to better articulate to others what her program was about and its benefits. Second, she wanted to figure out what grounded her in her work and possibly learn more about the way she was teaching so she could adjust (not necessarily improve or change) aspects of her teaching. Third, she wanted to tell her story about how she changed the way she thinks about physical education so that she could demonstrate to other physical educators that "if she could do it, so could they."

In that initial conversation, I was explicit about my intent. We briefly discussed key events and experiences that brought us to our current situations, as well as some initial thoughts about teaching physical education in this non-traditional way. We considered many different ideas, approaches and questions: What is the issue? Who is this for? What is the most important message? Kim's main concern was that it not be one of those programs that sat on the shelf in cello-wrap unopened or that it could be "cherry-picked" for parts that teachers dropped into their own programs but did nothing to change their perspectives. This called for a deeper understanding of what her program was about and what we meant by thinking differently about physical education. In the end, we both agreed that the focus needed to be on the teacher and the first step was to co-construct meaning on *teaching* a wellness-oriented, holistic, physical education curriculum.

Building Relationships

In traditional research paradigms, there is emphasis on minimizing the influence of the researcher on the environment or community being researched and maintaining objective distance between the researcher and participants. This dichotomous insider-outsider relationship was not appropriate in this inquiry because it would set up a power dynamic that is counterproductive to the goals of co-constructing knowledge. A collaborative, reciprocal and democratic relationship was imperative for Kim and me to be able to co-construct meaning. As a key ethic of this inquiry was grounded in action research, Herr and Anderson (2005) remind us that

> the researcher/researched relationship…comes from doing research *with* rather than
> *on*. Within a more collaborative research stance, decision making is more of a shared

process and insiders are part of the process in terms of assessing their own vulnerability as well as how to best return the data to the setting. (p. 123)

We met in the summer before fall classes to begin an adaptation of the *currere* process. It was important to Kim that we began this way, as she wanted to be in a less stressful environment and be able to focus on the present task without distraction. I agreed with this approach because I wanted to use the *currere* process to set the stage for building our co-researcher relationship. I also believed that the autobiographical process would provide a deeper understanding of how she came to teach in this way and thus a necessary piece to constructing meaning.

Much of the literature about *currere* focuses on its philosophical foundations and theoretical connections to education. Less is published about how the method of *currere* is lived. As such, I think it is important to share details about the events, timelines and steps we took to work through the stages of *currere*. I should note that the method of *currere* that we used was an adaptation of Pinar's method and I used Brown's (2007) doctoral work to design guiding questions.

Adapting the Method of *Currere*

At our first meeting, we reviewed the entire inquiry process and discussed scheduling for the stages of the *currere* process, my classroom observations, and one-on-one discussions for the fall. I also shared with Kim the process for the first stage of *currere*, the regressive. The regressive moment constitutes past lived experience, both personal and social, where the teacher re-enters the past in order to transform memory to the present (Pinar, 2004). I told her it is a time to think and write about significant people, places, and events that have shaped our ways of thinking about teaching physical education. I provided some guiding questions that help keep our writing in chronological order (Doerr, 2004). This ordering of events can be changed later but at this stage it is helpful for observing and recording relevant events.

- Think back to your early childhood and your experiences in and/or outside of school. What people, places, events do you remember? How did they make you feel? What was significant to you in shaping your teaching practice and your identity as a teacher?

- Think back to your adolescence and your experiences in and/or outside of school. What people, places, events do you remember? How did they make you feel? What was significant to you in shaping your teaching practice and your identity as a teacher?
- Think back to your time at university and your teacher education program. Who/what were the significant people, places, events in shaping your identity as a physical educator? Were there any significant experiences that influenced your way of teaching physical education?
- How would you describe your first few years of teaching? What sticks out in your mind—students, activities, program, colleagues? Are there any significant events that impacted your perspectives on teaching and/ or have shaped/is shaping your identity?

In this stage, you simply record your past observations without analysis, with the intent of "bringing the past to the present by printing it" (Pinar, 1994, p. 24). We spent two weeks remembering, feeling, and writing, and met again to share our stories—discussing our observations of significant people, events, places, emotions, and experiences that shaped our way of thinking about teaching physical education and have been instrumental in shaping our identities (as teacher, teacher educator, student and overall citizen in the world).

We next reviewed the process and guiding questions for the second stage, the progressive. In the progressive stage, one looks toward the future to what is not yet, to future possibilities. It was a visioning exercise that both of us found refreshing but somewhat unsettling, as we realized that it was something that we do not frequently do.

- Describe what is happening in your physical education classroom in 5, 10, 20 years from now? What are the students doing? What are the students like? What are you teaching? How are you teaching? What is the school like? Who are the key players in this scenario? How does it make you feel?
- Imagine you are about to receive recognition for something you have accomplished in teaching physical education. This is something you dreamed about before and now it has finally been achieved. What happened? How did you accomplish it? Who was involved? How does it make you feel?

One week later, we met to discuss our progressive stage writing and shared our observations about our identities as educators and teaching physical education in the future.

After three weeks spent on our autobiographical observations we began the third stage of *currere,* the analytical. In the analysis stage, the teacher examines past and present to create subjective space, ultimately asking the question: "How is the future present in the past, the past in the future and the present in both?" (Pinar, 2004, p. 37). Ultimately what you are looking for are themes from the snapshots of the self in the present, past, and future and any "complex multidimensional interrelations [you] can find within and between the photographs" (Doerr, 2004, p. 17). I provided some guiding questions for this stage as well but reminded Kim that these were just suggestions as to how to go about her analysis. Ultimately we were interested in answering the question: why are these experiences as they are?

- This stage is about looking at what you wrote/talked about in the previous stages and writing about/discussing that. This is a time to link the past and the future with your present. As you read what you have written about so far, what ideas show up over and over again? In what ways do these ideas ring as true for your past as for your present and your future?
- As you reread your writing, what parts are you drawn to? Which experiences are you most proud of? Which things do you wish you had done differently? Which experiences make you sad? What experiences make you angry? Which experiences leave you with mixed feelings?
- What decisions do you make today that are influenced by your past? How are decisions you make today influenced by what you hope for your future?
- As you read the writing, try to put your experiences into different categories or themes. What are the major themes of your stories about your past experiences and future vision? If you need a process to do this, here is one suggestion. Use note cards and put one word or two about each experience (just enough to jog your memory) on each card. Then sort the cards into categories that make sense to you. Record what categories you come up with.

We met again several weeks later to review our feelings and perceptions. It was a pivotal stage in our relationship and our longest discussion yet. We shared interpretations that were professional, personal, emotional, and cathartic, and revealed similarities that connected us as individuals on separate journeys yet now woven together.

At this point, we expected to move on to the fourth and final stage of *currere*—synthesis. However, we both felt that we had only scratched the surface of observing past, present, and future and analyzing the experiences we shared. We felt this would impact our ability to understand more fully what it meant regarding who she is as a teacher, how this impacted how she teaches, and its contribution to understanding what it means to teach a holistic, wellness-oriented approach to physical education. As Doerr (2004) explains, "over time we analyze our responses to experiences, we develop new meanings for our lives, which in turn produce new problems, new powers, new demands" (p. 184), thus the *currere* process needs ample space and time. As such, we paused and decided to continue with observing, recording, and analyzing throughout the semester.[1] So I began observing her class at the beginning of September, ensuring the classroom environment was established with my presence from the first class onward.

Living the Curriculum

My "observation" role alternated between participant observer and nonparticipant observer. Creswell (2005) refers to this as "a changing observational role…where researchers adapt their role to the situation" (p. 212). On the days that I was participant observer, I wrote reflectively after class, and as a nonparticipant observer I listened and watched from the periphery. I observed and participated in the class two to three times per week. The classes were 80 minutes long and I attended two separate sections of classes. There were 20 female students and one male student in the morning class, and 27 females and one male in the afternoon class. Each class consisted of a mix of grade 10, 11, and 12 students with the majority of students at the grade 10 level.

Kim and I continued to meet one-on-one for focused discussions, sharing pedagogical moments and reflections with the eventual goal of constructing meaning from past, present, and future critical events. While in traditional research one might call these interviews, it was important that these sessions were treated more as guided conversations between co-researchers because of the collaborative, dialectical, and democratic nature of action research. Lincoln and Guba (1985) explain that in this case, the co-researchers "create the data [together]…. Each influences the other, and the direction that the data gathering will take in the next moment is acutely dependent upon what data have already been collected, and in what manner" (p. 100). Stringer (2008) points out that "common approaches to interviewing based on extended lists of predefined questions are…inappropriate for the purpose of this type of research" (p. 58). Following the guiding philosophy of action research, we focused on Kim's perspective and allowed her to "describe, frame, and interpret events, issues, and other phenomena in [her] own terms" (Stringer, 2008, p. 58).

Both Kim and I kept reflective journals to record thoughts, significant events, and feelings. McKernan (1996) explains that journals are often used to "encourage description, interpretation, reflection and evaluation" (p. 84). Reflective writing provided a different way for us to express our experiences and observations, and analyze them in relation to the inquiry objectives. This ongoing reflective writing helped guide our conversations and helped identify emerging questions and themes that were helpful in co-constructing meaning about a wellness curriculum. "Meaning," Schutz tells us, "does not lie in experience. Rather, those experiences are meaningful which are grasped reflectively" (as cited in Grumet, 1987, p. 322).

Wisdom, *Currere,* and Action Research[2]

When I began this inquiry, I knew that curriculum reform in physical education was partially dependent on how physical educators understand curriculum. Further, I was interested in a more holistic, wellness-oriented approach that was grounded in wisdom traditions and existential perspectives, and an understanding of curriculum as *currere.* Thus, I chose to work with a physical education teacher who had designed a "holistic health" course within her physical education department. While I assumed that she did not know much about curriculum theory, it was clear to me that something had taken place for this teacher to precipitate her looking at teaching physical education in a different way. I was not necessarily interested in the technical aspects of the course, as I knew a copy of the curriculum document would satisfy this aspect. I was more interested in who she was as a teacher, what it meant to teach in a wellness-oriented way, and how the curriculum was lived. This is a departure from how physical education typically understands "practice" (related to techne), which is guided by preconceived activities and standards of performance. The idea of teaching as "a way of being" allows us to consider practice differently, as *phronesis*—knowledge from the practical disciplines that is dialectical in thought and action and grounded in a "moral disposition to act truly and justly" (Carr & Kemmis, 1986, p. 33).

To understand the significance of the distinction between *techne* and *phronesis* for the field of physical education, it is necessary to trace these philosophical concepts back to Aristotle. Although there are subsequent philosophers[3] who have explored the relations between technical and practical reason, I will be limiting this discussion to Aristotelian analysis.

While the focus of this discussion is on "nontheoretical" forms of knowledge, it is important to distinguish this practical side of knowledge from theoretical knowledge. Aristotle believed that theoretical knowledge, *episteme*, was "neither practical nor productive" (Dunne, 1993, p. 237). Theoretical activity was based in contemplation with its *telos* being the "attainment of knowledge for its own sake" (Carr & Kemmis, 1986, p. 238). The highest level of theoretical knowledge is the philosophical wisdom of *sophia*, which "was of the greatest difficulty—in that it was furthest from the senses—and at the same time it was the most perspicuous (and hence teachable)—in that it reached the highest level of intelligibility in things" (Dunne, 1993, p. 238). Both *sophia* and *theoria* (universal knowledge) were specifically distinguished from knowledge of a productive and practical nature, techne and phronesis. Hanley (1998) further explains, theoria "is concerned with the question of why, and the answer to this question does not necessarily have practical consequences" (p. 3).

Inquiry and knowledge associated with what Aristotle classed in the productive disciplines was called *poietike*. The end disposition of techne is *poiesis*, an "activity which is designed to bring about, and which terminates in, a product or outcome that is separable from it and provides it with its end" (Dunne, 1993, p. 244). Carr and Kemmis (1986) refer to this as "instrumental reasoning"—"as 'making action'…which is evident in craft or skill knowledge" (p. 32). Knowledge from the practical disciplines is called *phronesis* with its end disposition, *praxis*, translating into "doing action." Phronesis is dialectical in thought and action, and is grounded in a "moral disposition to act truly and justly" (Carr & Kemmis, 1986, p. 33). According to Dunne (1993), phronesis "characterizes a person who knows how to live well (*eu zen*)" (p. 244). Aristotle makes a very specific distinction between these two types of activity in that phronesis is "the reasoned state of capacity to act" and techne is "the reasoned state of capacity to make" (Aristotle, as cited in Dunne, 1993, p. 244).

Considering curriculum as *currere* and teaching as a way of being (with grounding in phronesis) laid the groundwork to conducting an inquiry into what it means to teach a wellness approach to physical education. However, the challenge was that the *way* I went about conducting this inquiry to construct this meaning with a teacher in the field had to also reflect and honor the principles of wisdom, a *currere* perspective, and the existential lens that distinguishes "the act of teaching from *being* a teacher" (Feldman, 2009, p. 381). The *complicated conversation* that resulted was a merging of philosophies—*currere*, wisdom traditions, existential perspectives (primarily from Maxine Greene), and the concept of *action research as an ethos* to form a new way of doing and living research—wisdom-guided inquiry.

One may argue that wisdom-guided inquiry is not a merging of philosophies; rather it is that these philosophies need each other when addressing what it means to teach in this way. Without looking at curriculum as *currere*—active, subjective, social, a conversation about our lives and how we live them—there would be no need to explore what it means to teach a wellness-oriented approach grounded in wisdom traditions. Because *currere* is about the educational experience and how we live our lives, it does not make sense to look at what is going on in a classroom from the technical, traditional way of looking at teaching practice, and thus the focus on teaching as a way of being. So not only are the phenomenological and existential roots of *currere* important here but specifically the existential concepts of the emergence of self, dialectical freedom, and situatedness. Inherent in the statement "teaching as a way of being" is this notion of there being *a way*.

Wisdom traditions guide us to re-examine our world from a point of view that demands consciousness, mindfulness, a connection between the mind and heart. Wisdom cannot be accumulated in the epistemological sense. Wisdom is about a way of being in relation to others and the cosmos, thus more than epistemological knowledge but also ontological, axiological, and cosmological. The defining term for all wisdom traditions is *the Way*, where we are to focus on the very manner of our living. Wisdom traditions help us to challenge our assumptions about how we conduct ourselves in this world, to "see" the origins of our problems, to name our struggles for what they are (not what they are supposed to be), and encourage the stillness that is needed to recover the mind-body-spirit connection that is part of our primary existence. This not only points to how we go about helping students learn how to live their own lives of wellness; but wisdom's response to this issue is that starting with the self, as teachers we must begin to ask ourselves how the very manner of our living affects our students' health and wellbeing. Park (1996) explains,

> The primary resource you have as a teacher is your self, your whole self, mind and spirit and body, and unless you are willing to teach with your whole self, with everything you have, you are not really going to teach at all. (p. 7)

In many Indigenous traditions, ways of knowing are connected to actions—there is no meaning without a unity between words and action. So too is our way of co-constructing meaning in this inquiry. So far, we have a cognitive understanding about a *way of being* on the journey of life and that is what will remain unless we experience, do, move, act, and relate. Without action, knowledge is incomplete. Therefore, to embark upon an inquiry with a teacher who is challenging traditional curriculum views, an underlying vision from wisdom traditions, *currere* and existentialism, and attempting to co-create knowledge (ontological, epistemological, axiological and cosmological),[4] one needs to do more than observe to understand. Hence, action research has a valuable contribution to make to this mode of inquiry. Action research is an ethos that guides researchers in an inquiry process that calls attention to "the specific relational organization of one's living conditions…ones which can[not] be predetermined and established as fixed and prescriptive methods" (Sumara & Carson, 1997, p. xvi). Action research takes into consideration the pathway it takes to come to a conclusion, not just in a methodological sense, but also in a relational way where the connections between the research, participants, and the inquiry subject are complicated (Sumara & Carson, 1997). In other words, research about wellness that is grounded in wisdom, with a teacher who has a certain existential and phenomenological way of being, must be situated within a particular ethos that is reflective, relational, reciprocal, participatory, emancipatory, and democratizing. *Action research as an ethos* provides an opportunity for the researcher and participant(s) to enter into a collaborative relationship that respects the synchronic nature of knowledge creation and application (Greenwood & Levin, 2007).

The Tensions of Connecting *Currere* and Action Research

I want to briefly discuss the nature of how I came to live (not just embody) and understand this inquiry process as being unique. As those closest to me will attest, I struggled on how to bring *currere* and action research together in this inquiry. The struggles I faced as a researcher to conduct this inquiry were related to the connectivity between my own *currere* processes and Kim's, as well as being able to use these moments to co-construct meaning in a dynamic, dialogical, collaborative way. My own *currere* understandings were central to situating me in this inquiry and I was careful in how and when I presented my stories, if at all. I would share my *currere* moments only if I was also able to maintain the collaborative relationship. Listening, discussing, and interacting in the co-researcher relationship—I was constantly revisiting regressive and progressive moments and analyzing as she was speaking and doing—in order to re-write and synthesize the present moment. In essence, she was doing the same. We would then share and discuss further, and together synthesize into the whole. This was the ongoing action research piece of co-constructing meaning. We were constantly building upon moments.

My *currere* process, this self-analytical, autobiographical way of thinking about myself and my field—who I am and how I am situated in relation to others (collectively, historically, politically, socially, culturally)—is in itself a way of being, a way of inquiring. I was constantly circling dynamically in a temporal nonlinearity, interacting and connecting with Kim and revisiting my own story as a way to actively understand teaching in a way that helps students live well. As I lived the curriculum with Kim and listened to stories from her own *currere*, I was constantly reviewing my own story in relation to hers. This influenced how I listened to what she had to say and how I contemplated and continually reconsidered the inquiry. This is the unique character of this inquiry—the connectivity between Kim and myself and the intersection of our *currere* experiences. It was a physically, emotionally, spiritually, and mentally involved process that extends beyond the personal and intimate nature of the individual *currere* processes to a collaborative endeavor.

This dynamic weaving and flow of *currere* processes has *a way* to it, each circle or spiral, each synthetical moment is noticed. Understanding that our mindful ways of being impact our synthetical moments, we were presently aware and sought to understand how these moments are connected to ourselves, others, and the natural world. Connecting *currere* and action research is a "dialogical co-creating unity between self and other" (Smith, 2013, p. 49) (individually and collectively)—this is the nature of wisdom-guided inquiry and living a curriculum of wellness.

· 2 ·

CONNECTING THEORETICAL PERSPECTIVES TO A CURRICULUM OF WELLNESS

I am who I am not yet.

— Maxine Greene, 1996

Before I began my scholarly journey, I had started to challenge my own philosophy of teaching physical education because students were becoming more and more disengaged in my sport technique–focused program (Kirk, 2010). I began envisioning a physical education whereupon graduation my students were able to take care of themselves and others—physically, emotionally, mentally, and spiritually. I realized that focusing on the body without a connection to mind and spirit actually resulted in individual and collective ways of being that were unhealthy, not well. But to promote programming that supports non-Cartesian, nondualistic thinking is difficult, as our individual and collective identities with the field of physical education are tightly wound within this way of knowing. I wondered if it was worth continuing on this path and I paused for a moment to contemplate my next step within a field I was so passionate about.

Early in my academic career, I was introduced to Maxine Greene, one of the most significant educational philosophers of our time. I was amazed at how even at her then age of 92, her contribution to the field of education was and still is not complete. "Her own sense of incompletion," explains Pinar

(2007), "of what is not yet but can be, inspires us to work for a future we can only imagine now" (p. 151). Vision, imagination, and inspiration—she had my attention. I felt somewhat comforted, as some of my previous colleagues had said I was naïve and misguided by ideas that were just not possible. Maxine Greene's educational vision prompted me to further philosophize about physical education reform and (re)consider the "power of the possible," to "what is not yet." Her words inspired me to forge ahead with the vision for physical education reform where students' overall wellness—body, mind, and spirit—was the priority, not sport technique and movement skills.

This chapter outlines key concepts in curriculum theory that are important for the discussion about a curriculum of wellness and physical education reform. Kirk (2013) asks "whether physical education has a future in the twenty-first century" (p. 221). I approach the notion of physical education curriculum from a reconceptualist view and utilize the philosophical perspectives of Maxine Greene, curriculum as *currere*, wisdom traditions, and action research as an ethos to inform and inspire my work on physical education reform.

In this chapter, I will outline and explore four of Maxine Greene's existential concepts—wide-awakeness, mindfulness, teacher as stranger, and dialectical freedom—in relation to physical education, teachers, and teaching. Next, I will explain curriculum as *currere* and make the key point that this concept is one of the missing components in physical education. I will also provide a review of wisdom traditions including a brief genealogy, background, and description of key characteristics and discuss how wisdom can better inform physical education curriculum. Finally, I will examine *action research as an ethos* and its importance to working collaboratively with teachers.

Perspectives from Maxine Greene

Wide-Awakeness and Mindfulness

Greene (1978) urges both teachers and students to become wide-awake, which she defines as "a plane of consciousness of highest tension originating in an attitude of full attention to life and its requirements" (p. 42). This "wakeful presence" is needed to connect body-mind-spirit and prevents us from "spinning out in thought"—where we can "discover newness, our most trustworthy ground and support" (Welwood, 1992, p. xxiii). Wide-awakeness allows us to "find a space for allowing multiple perspectives" (Slattery & Dees, 1998, p. 50) and perhaps in the physical education world will help teachers see how physical education's fundamental philosophy of body-as-object (Tinning, 2004; Colquhoun, 1990) has created a culture that does not nurture the wholeness of living with which children are born.

Being "wide-awake" is particularly important for teachers, as being open to multiple perspectives allows for the reflexivity and creative reflection that is needed to "shift our consciousness (of ourselves, of others, of the nature of thoughts, feelings, professional practices, etc.)" (Winter, 2003, p. 150). This type of reflectiveness enables people to pay "full attention to life" and encourages individuals to engage with others creatively and imaginatively. It promotes a humanistic dialogue about "what it is to be human, to grow, to be" (Greene, 1977, p. 123) and "once this occurs, new perspectives will open up—perspectives on the past, on cumulative meanings, on future possibilities" (p. 123).

Mindfulness and wide-awakeness are intricately related to subjectivity and primordial consciousness. We must mindfully educate and find ways for our students to pay attention to what Freire calls "background awareness"—that which naturally exists within the human body before codification (Greene, 1971). Greene (1984a) believes that by nurturing mindfulness, we empower students to be critically conscious of themselves and others. This is particularly important in the challenges of the information age with the "overabundance of fragmented information" and the "onslaught of slogans and images and pieties" (p. 293). When we become distracted, we lose our ability to be present and succumb to the fast-paced swirling of our materialistic world. Mindfulness is one way to help prevent spinning out of control individually and collectively, to stop the steady decline of health of people and the planet, and to connect body, mind, and spirit.

Teacher as Stranger and Teacher Identity

Based on my own experience, I believe that teacher as stranger is one of the most important of Greene's themes for physical educators. Teacher as stranger begins to address how we form our collective and individual identities. We define our own individual identities but are also influenced by perceptions and encounters with the collective. This means that identity is formed in a dynamic and dialectical way. Identity is temporal, spatial, relational, and embodied in nature, and as such, it can never be static. Identity formation is an active, continuous, flowing process that positions the individual in relation to others, events, encounters, context, orientation, and environment. Although identity formation is active, there is a tendency to want to hold on to things as time and space change around us. I believe this can be a source of despair and hopelessness, leading to feelings of low self-worth and affecting overall health and wellbeing. While not easy, if we could embrace the flowing nature of our identities, be comfortable here and there, accept the role as stranger, perhaps this would challenge the "overdominance culture" (Kwan, 2008) that exists within the empirically based, sport-focused discourse in physical education. When there is an overdominance of identification within a culture, it is difficult to maintain or propose new ways of knowing, thinking, doing, and being.

This tension between collective and individual identity is a core issue that explains why the physical education environment has not changed over the past 50 years. My identity as a physical educator, for example, was relational to the mentors and colleagues who held sport in highest regard as a curricular focus. Of course, my background as an athlete also contributed to my identity as a physical education teacher who valued sport performance, measurement, and a certain physique. As time progressed, I had different life experiences and relationships that changed my identity as a physical educator. But this shift in my identity formation only happened because I was able to step back and challenge my own assumptions, and interrogate the collective life history of my field. Encouraging physical educators to accept the role of "teacher as stranger" may provide opportunities for present and future change.

Dialectical Freedom

Greene's desire to explore other ways of seeing, other ways of being in the world is grounded in her conceptualization of freedom. Her interest is in "human freedom, in the capacity to surpass the given and to look at things as if they could be otherwise" (Greene, 1988, p. 3). This builds on what Dewey said about freedom: "we are free not because of what we statically are, but in so far as we are becoming different from what we have been" (Dewey, as cited in Greene, 1988, p. 3). Greene also believes that freedom is situated, in other words, free activity is defined according to our "acceptance of our defining situation" (p. 7).

Adding to the concepts of humanness and situatedness is that freedom is dialectical. The world can be understood as composed of dichotomies that are intertwined and interconnected. It is not either/or; it is different degrees of both and the whole range in between based on context and intention. Every situation is dialectical in that there is always a relationship between at least two things: subject–object, individual–environment, self–society, outsider–community. Although these seem to be two poles, they are still connected on the same spectrum, which assumes a type of mediation, "something that occurs between nature and culture, work and action, technologies and human minds" (Greene, 1988, p. 8). This tension is always present yet it cannot be overcome by triumph by one side or the other, nor can it be resolved "in some perfect synthesis or harmony" (p. 8). The point is, freedom is being able to understand the ambiguities, the layers of determinateness of our lives. Freedom is connected to human consciousness, which "involves the capacity to pose questions to the world, to reflect on what is presented in experience" (p. 21). In education, the dialectic teaching-learning environment involves a mutual quest for multiple perspectives, "each person reaches out from his/her own ground toward what might be, should be, is not yet" (p. 21).

This dialectic environment is fundamental to the field of education, and in this case, physical education, because it involves teachers understanding their freedom, recognizing the limitations of freedom, and acknowledging their relationship with others (especially students) and their ability to act responsibly towards themselves and others. It requires one to be aware of the lived situation (which is tempered by the backdrop of our own life histories and that of our collective life history) and how it is interpreted against the possibilities for action. As Greene (1988) says, "this means that one's 'reality,' rather than being fixed and predefined, is a perpetual emergent, becoming increasingly multiplex, as more perspectives are taken, more texts are opened" (p. 23).

Reconceptualizing Curriculum

Greene's work and passion inspired me to look in directions I likely would not have considered in the area of health and physical education. Her ideas in "Curriculum and Consciousness" (1971), her books and other collected works, provided a basis for me to begin my research journey with a new lens—a willingness to see the world from multiple perspectives, to be "wide-awake" to the possibilities, to question, to move beyond. It was at this point I learned about the reconceptualization of curriculum studies. I believe that physical education's dominant curriculum orientation foundation is primarily traditional, as there is evidence of technical rationality driving curriculum development. It was my experience as a curriculum manager at the Ministry of Education in Alberta, Canada, and as a physical educator in junior and high school programs in British Columbia, that most activities and behaviors were measured and quantified (even the affective objectives). I was not aware that there was a reconceptualization of curriculum, as my reality was a predominately sport performance–based curriculum. To more fully understand the reconceptualist movement, I will provide a brief background of the key events.

Against the backdrop of modernity and the resistance from those who support a technical Tyler Rationale, postmodernism provided an avenue for education to understand curriculum in a different way. Within that postmodern perspective, there was a paradigm shift in the 1970s from a "primary and practical interest in the *development* of curriculum to a theoretical and practical interest in *understanding* curriculum (Pinar, Reynolds, Slattery & Taubman, 2004, p. 187). One of the key catalysts of this paradigm shift, where conceptually and methodologically the field of curriculum studies began its reconceptualization, was Schwab's (1970) declaration that "the field is moribund. It is unable, by its present methods and principles, to continue and contribute significantly to the advancement of education" (as cited in Pinar et al., 2004, p. 193).

As Pinar and colleagues (2004) explain, the reason for this need for change in the early 1970s was about meaning, not performance. The Tyler Rationale that focuses on "means-end" education was met with confusion by educators, "thereby making it impossible to reach the end for which the means were devised" (Silberman, 1970, as cited in Pinar et al., 2004, p. 188). A more humanistic way of education began to dominate the discussion within curriculum studies.

Self-actualization, originally highlighted by psychologist Abraham Maslow, represented one form of humanistic development that influenced curriculum development to be more "humane." Influenced by Arthur Foshay, a more humanistic approach included such concepts as

> persons as holistic and in a state of becoming or growing, the necessity of interaction with the environment for learning and knowledge creation, the importance of dialogue for both the exchange and growth of knowledge, and the centrality of acknowledging and fostering individuality. (Pinar et al., 2004, p. 190)

Schwab's influence further strengthened the reconceptualist movement when he emphasized thinking about *particular* students (not generic) in the local context—the human beings who are actually in front of you with all their unique, individual characteristics (Pinar et al., 2004, p. 197).

Pinar (1978/2004; Giroux, Penna, & Pinar, 1981) categorizes the curriculum field into three perspectives: traditional, conceptual-empirical, and reconceptualist. Traditional curriculum theorists identify most closely with Tyler and prioritize functional knowledge, technical rationality, and "transmission forms of instruction" (Giroux, Penna, & Pinar, 1981, p. 14). Conceptual-empirical perspectives are characterized by logic and scientifically based investigation where hypotheses are tested methodically such as is done by social scientists. A focus on the scientific method often precludes the acceptance of other ways of knowing (e.g., literature, aesthetics, arts) and "facts are considered as clearly separable from values" (Giroux, Penna, & Pinar, 1981, p. 14). The reconceptualist perspective accepts that curriculum is political and situated historically (Pinar, 1978/2004). Its hermeneutic theme emphasizes subjectivity, autobiographical, phenomenological, existential experience, and a "centrality of intentionality to understanding human action" (Giroux, Penna, & Pinar, 1981, p. 14). Furthermore, reconceptualists study "matters of temporality, transcendence, consciousness and politics" (Pinar, 1975, p. xiii), and endeavor to understand the educational experience.

Curriculum conversations in physical education have taken place primarily from a traditionalist perspective, although some conceptual-empiricist perspectives have made their way into the physical education literature as well. As discussed by Kirk (1993), whether we consider Jewett and Mullan's (1977) Purpose-Process-Curriculum Framework, Hellison's (1985) socio-cultural considerations, Siedentop, Mand, and Taggart's (1986) emphasis on observable behavioral objectives and systemic procedures, or Rink's (1985) goal-oriented approach, the commonality among these perspectives is that curriculum is still viewed as something to be *applied* (on)to the "one-size-fits-all" student, a collection of technical end goals of overt performance that are measurable against preconceived standards, and that there is a separation between knowledge, subjectivity, and culture (Pinar, 2004).

Although many curriculum scholars have called for those in the education field to engage in theorizing (e.g., Ted Aoki, Dwayne Huebner, William Pinar, Madeleine Grumet, William Schubert, Janet Miller), it is rare to see dialogue in the physical education community about curriculum theory (with the exception of such scholars as Ann Jewett, Linda Bain, Richard Tinning, Doune Macdonald, David Kirk). A reconceptualized understanding of curriculum has yet to gain much momentum in physical education and I suggest that the powerful influence of science and sport will continue to undermine efforts to look at physical education beyond the technicist orientation. Thinking or theorizing about curriculum in physical education usually takes the form of discussion about curriculum design, development, and implementation within the narrow context of the gymnasium, field, or other school physical activity space. Schubert (2009) reminds us of Pinar's emphasis on *understanding* curriculum, "in contrast with curriculum development that focuses on efficient design for implementing institutional purposes" (p. 137). He further delineates that "*understanding* invokes an inclusiveness in curriculum studies of a wide range of scholarship devoted to understanding cultural phenomena that shape who and what human beings become within or apart from schooling" (p. 137). Macdonald et al. (2002) also remind physical education researchers about theoretical perspectives and ensuring theory connections are made to political, economic, and cultural issues, data collection, as well as avoiding theoretical fads.

In a time where the future of physical education is under scrutiny, I believe it is time for the field of physical education "to do some philosophy" (Greene, 1973, p. 7), step back to see the bigger picture, and ask the broader question about what grounds the field in how it looks at curriculum. We should begin to have the *complicated conversation* about what constitutes knowledge and knowing in physical education and what curriculum is in relation to our students, community, and the world.

Pinar (1978/2004) explains, "what is necessary is a fundamental reconceptualization of what curriculum is, how it functions, and how it might function in emancipatory ways" (p. 154). While the reconceptualist movement began in the early 1970s, there has been little discussion about it in the field of physical education. Perhaps my generation of physical education scholars is the "generation of scholars sympathetic to reconceptualist thinking" (Graham, 1992, p. 40), and although it is two decades since Graham (1992) originally claimed that "reconceptualism still represents one of the best hopes for keeping the human factor alive in education" (p. 40), I believe this is true for physical education today.

Accordingly, reconceptualization is the direction I decided to follow— maintaining the human element, understanding curriculum as "organismic rather than mechanistic" (Pinar & Grumet, 1976, p. 32), and looking at physical education beyond "scientific functionalism" and "utilitarian knowledge" (Devis-Devis & Sparkes, 1999, p. 148) where knowledge is accepted for its extrinsic nature (i.e., promoting elite performance, discipline, conformity, academics, employment). As Grumet (Pinar & Grumet, 1976) further explains,

> The traditional view, reflected in the methodology of the social sciences, describes human development as a sum of its parts, organized in an incremental hierarchy leading to resolution realized in operational competencies.... In contrast, the form of

the reconceptualist is horizontal, rather than vertical, its energy moving outward and inward rather than upward in a linear trajectory. The form is at once centripetal and centrifugal. Its center is a crossing point where the lines of energy intersect: lines of force drawn into form by the opposition and tension of the dialectic, id/ego, subjectivity/objectivity, community/individuality, consciousness/matter. (p. 33)

Curriculum as *Currere*

With my exploration of Greene's work and my commitment to a reconceptualized physical education curriculum as being critical to breaking the cycle of recycled ideas, I was intrigued about the origins and etymology of the term "curriculum." The Latin infinitive form of curriculum, *currere*, means "the running of the course." How apropos that with my background as a track-and-field athlete and physical education teacher, that *curriculum* was associated with a Roman chariot track and something active. Considering curriculum in this manner disrupted my traditional, taken-for-granted view of curriculum as a document outlining the set of learning outcomes that guide classroom activities. Instead of Goodson's (1997) interpretation of *currere* (n.)—a course to be followed or presented—the Latin infinitive form of *currere* (v.) means curriculum becomes active, subjective, social, a conversation about our lives and how we live them (Pinar, 2012). Understanding curriculum as *currere* provides an alternate outlook about teaching physical education where we understand that our *being* cannot be separated from the world, and we take into account our location—in temporal, spatial, and embodied form—in history and culture. Pinar (Pinar & Grumet, 1976) further explains:

> Curriculum reconceptualized is *currere*; it is not the course to be run, or the artifacts employed in the running of the course; it is the running of the course. The course most broadly is our lives, in schools and out, and the running, is our experiences of our lives. Because our lives tend to be progressive, we say that we evolve. This evolution is education; it is the synthesis of cognitive and psychosocial development. (p. 18)

Grumet (1980) refers to curriculum as *currere* as "the journey of life," an "exploration of educational experience" (Pinar & Grumet, 1976, p. 35). I am not suggesting that physical education abandon its epistemological ways of knowing. I am merely recognizing that our field is in need of what Pinar (2004) refers to as "a more complicated conversation" (p. 9) where we engage in "frank and ongoing self-criticism…with our academic subjects, our students and ourselves" (p. 9).

This means that physical education's epistemological definition of knowledge will also require an ontological, axiological, and cosmological foundation.

Doerr (2004) explains that with *currere*, the focus shifts from the prescriptive to understanding, where the individual experiencing the curriculum is the focus. She reiterates Pinar's perspective that *currere* encourages an

> awakening to the indifference that is so often promulgated in schools, where students absorb the reality the schools construct.... Pinar believes the habits and compliance that schools produce can be shaken up by allowing students to address questions that increase awareness of how they live within their worlds. (p. 9)

This touches on Camus's *The Plague* when Tarrou uses the retelling of the past to understand how he has reconstituted his world, developed his own traditions, and revealed context for his future. This attempt to describe life "in the context of human-being-within-the-world" (Doerr, 2004, p. 9) is what Pinar is advocating for with *currere*.

Currere draws from an ontological foundation in humanistic philosophy, phenomenology, and existentialism (primarily the dialectic between individuals and their situation) (Pinar & Grumet, 1976, p. 35). *Currere* considers a reciprocal relationship between subjectivity and objectivity, "each constituting each other" (p. 36). Grumet explains that "to talk of education as the dialogue of a man and his world is not to break down this complex interaction into separate parts, subjecting each to a distinct isolated analysis" and that "approaches to curriculum are too often drawn to one pole of the dialectic or the other" (p. 36). Dualism of body-mind is an example of this conflict, and physical education's dominant discourse usually rests at the pole of body-as-object, body-as-machine. This view of the body can be traced back to the Cartesian discourse of the body, where body and mind are considered separate, and technical and scientific ways of knowing are emphasized over social and interpretive knowledge (Fitzclarence & Tinning, 1990). Resisting rest at one pole of the dialectic or the other, allowing the polarities to "dissolve into reciprocity" (Pinar & Grumet, 1976, p. 36) allows us to consider

> the human as an embodied experiencer and suggests (perhaps demands) an integration of those aspects that are objectively accessible with those that are subjectively experienced. It allows us to focus not only on the movement of the human but also on the human moving. (Rintala, 1991, p. 262)

This implies that when (re)designing curriculum, the educational experience of the individual should be consulted and the ambiguity of nonduality accepted. Perhaps then we will be able to negotiate beyond a mechanistic, measured, standardized, skill-production approach to physical education to one that also considers the human experience in relation to one's world.

This human experience in relation to one's world is an existential phenomenological notion that is referring to the situatedness of the individual or the dialectic of the individual to one's situation. Again, what is important here is not the analysis of the situation as a cause of the individual's experience or vice versa, but *understanding* the individual's experience. This means that research in physical education that produces lists of empirically obtained health or sport skill measures as a basis to determine curriculum or program effectiveness presents a depersonalized and fragmented notion of the educational experience. Implementing a new curriculum or program without understanding the experience of the individuals participating in it may provide an explanation as to why physical education curriculum has had little impact on long-term healthy active living habits (Kirk, 2013). *Currere* encourages "a return to the experience of the individual" (Pinar & Grumet, 1976, p. 45) and suggests that we "study both the individual's subjectivity and the impact of his social milieu upon it" (p. 45). Further, *currere* not only is interested in the impact of milieu but the political present and subjective past synchronously (Pinar & Grumet, 1976).

The existential phenomenological foundations of *currere* not only draw attention to an individual's subjectivity and connections to the greater social, political, and historical context, but also emphasize regressive and progressive analysis to be able to "re-write" (synthesize) the present. This process requires individuals to stop and pay attention. This type of stillness or meditative practice can result in an "emerging awareness that so many of the pedagogical problems that preoccupy us as teachers can be, and in fact need to be, reinterpreted" (Smith, 2008b, p. 29). Smith (2008b) further explains,

> meditation affords the possibility of seeing and naming what is going on in the pedagogical situation for what it is, not for what it is supposed to be according to the hyperbolized prescriptions of state and nation.... This gaining of the freedom to see the world as it actually is is the deepest meaning of wisdom. (p. 29)

Wisdom Traditions

In the following, I will present a brief overview of my understanding of wisdom traditions. My purpose is not to provide a detailed description and explanation of the numerous traditions but to present a brief genealogical overview of the notion of wisdom and a few examples of wisdom traditions from around the world.

Evidence of the notion of wisdom can be found in many cultures and spiritual traditions worldwide. Traditional Christian views are complex and include both Hebraic and Hellenic understandings from the New Testament. Hebraism focused on the *revealed* truth, whereas Hellenic canon is interested in a state of being (Robinson, 1990). With these varying perspectives, Christianity has had somewhat of a divided history. Some of this division comes from the differing views of Plato, Socrates, and Aristotle. Platonic writings outline wisdom as *sophia*, wisdom as *phronesis*, and wisdom as *episteme*. Wisdom as *sophia* refers to "the special gift of the philosopher and of those in general who have devoted themselves to a contemplative life in pursuit of truth" (Robinson, 1990, p. 14). Wisdom as *phronesis* is "the 'practical wisdom' of the statesman and lawgiver, the wisdom that locates the prudent course of action and resists the urgings of the passions and the deceptions of the senses" (p. 14). Wisdom as *episteme* can be thought of as the "form of scientific knowledge developed in those who know the nature of things and the principles governing their behaviour" (p. 14).

The Socratic notion of wisdom introduces a division between mental skills and wisdom: "Wise men may be illiterate, and the utterly unwise may be adept and accomplished" (p. 14). Socrates did not trust knowledge in its perceptual form or empirical inquiry. He believed that "the wisdom-loving person—the *philos-sophia*—is one who searches for the timeless and unchanging truths, never content with the shifting phenomena of the material world" (Robinson, 1990, p. 15).

Aristotle may have presented the first psychological and naturalistic perspective related to wisdom. He rejected previous views that separated the body from the soul and that wisdom is "life lived in a certain way" (Robinson, 1990, p. 16). The character of the person and his or her disposition (hexis) was the key consideration regarding wisdom for Aristotle. "To be wise is...to have passions and desires that are rightly disposed, such that one's deliberated choice (*prohairesis*) is always of that which promotes the flourishing of one's human and humanizing attributes" (Robinson, 1990, p. 17). While there is much variation in the notion of wisdom throughout Christian teachings, there seems to be one commonality: "to be wise is to be touched by the divine wisdom that conveys timeless and boundless verities" (Robinson, 1990, p. 20).

Asian and Indigenous wisdom traditions are also rich with history, and form another part of the genealogy of wisdom traditions. For example,

Buddhism is based on the teachings of Siddhartha Gautama (Buddha), who was born in the sixth century BCE. Buddhist wisdom is described as the understanding of four noble truths: (i) life means suffering; (ii) the origin of suffering is attachment; (iii) the cessation of suffering is attainable; (iv) the path to end suffering is achieved through the practice of mindfulness (Butler, 2011).

Confucianism was developed from the teachings of Chinese philosopher Confucius (K'ung Fu Tzu), who was born in 551 BCE. The main idea behind the tradition of Confucianism is the cultivation of virtue and development of moral perfection (Lai, 2008). Confucianism focuses on the following values: Li (ritual, propriety, etiquette); Hsiao (love within family); Yi (righteousness); Xin (honesty and trustworthiness); Jen (benevolence, humaneness towards others); and Chung (loyalty to the state) (Confucianism, n.d.).

Taoism originated in China from two main philosophers: Lao Tzu (believed to have lived between sixth and third century BCE) and Chuang Tzu (369–286 BCE). Tao means "the path" or "the way"—"living in concordance with the unity of the universe…in harmony with all others, with the environment and with one's self. It is to live in synchronicity with processes, and to be completely authentic, sincere, natural and innocent" (Dale, 2006, p. 2).

The wisdom from the many Indigenous cultures worldwide has similar themes, including relationships between individuals, the interconnectedness of everything, and honoring the ways of the past (cultural traditions) to guide our present and future (Share the World, 2011; Jamieson, 2011). Through his stories about the Navajo, Toelken (1976) explains how, for many Indigenous cultures, spirituality is "viewed as embodying the reciprocal relationships between people and the sacred *processes* going on in the world" (p. 14). For the Navajo, everything is related to health. In the Western world, health is normally thought in terms of medical issues. Whereas the Navajo believe that one must visit a spiritual leader to "reestablish his relationship with the rhythms of nature…the medicine may cure the symptoms, but it won't cure you" (Toelken, 1976, p. 15). They rely on this reciprocal relationship and circular pattern of life to guide the "singer" in how to use medicinal materials and put you back in the natural cycle. This notion of reciprocation is an example of a way of living life, a mindful way of being *in* the world. This is consistent with many of the wisdom traditions and common when tracing the origins of wisdom.

There is considerable literature that addresses the broader area of individual and community health and outlines the types of Indigenous perspectives that illustrate living life in a healthful way. According to Stewart (2007, as cited in Hill, 2009), Indigenous practices that help heal and address wellbeing include: storytelling, advice from Elders, interconnectedness with family and community, healing circles and ceremony. In a study of Australian Aborigines' health, Thompson and Gifford (2000) speak about "the maintenance of meaningful connections to family, the land, the past and future, all of which are important for health and wellbeing" (p. 1458). Kirby (2007) points to a "lack of culturally relevant opportunities" (p. 12) in a Canadian study of northern-rural Aboriginal community members' physical activity involvement. The author further explains how modernization has shifted traditional ways of living to Western, efficiency-based practices that tend to promote sedentary lifestyle behaviors. This research suggests that by focusing on cultural traditions and reconnecting to the land, physical activity can become a part of everyday life. This suggestion is "consistent with a wholistic approach to healthy living that is embraced by many members of the Aboriginal community" (p. 18)[1] and is an example of a wisdom response to calls for healthy living.

Smith (2013) outlines the difficulty in summarizing all wisdom traditions into one succinct description,

> What is meant by the term "Wisdom Traditions" when it is used in the context of appealing to wisdom as a source for pedagogical, indeed social and cultural insight? The question pulls us into some very murky water, as issues arise regarding commensurability of meaning across massive differences of historical and geographical experience. (p. 52)

After many years of scholarship in this area, Smith (2013) offers several characteristics of wisdom traditions and their connections to the "practice of pedagogical wisdom," including: (i) wisdom acknowledges the inherent unity of birth and death, (ii) wisdom contradicts values of power by revealing the paradoxical nature of experience, (iii) wisdom fractures the temporal enframing of conventional interpretation, (iv) wisdom understands the natural world as pedagogical, and (v) wisdom honors the intermingling of implicate and explicate orders.

One other overarching principle of wisdom traditions is the notion that there is a *Way* to life—consciousness, mindfulness, and a connection between the mind, body, and heart. It requires the practice of stillness, and in this active, ongoing practice, we become presently aware of ourselves and others. These are matters of action and relationality that are also significant to action research.

Action Research

Susan Noffke (2009) says that action research has many purposes, and its multidimensional nature "offers a way to understand and thereby use action research as a means not solely for knowledge generation...but for personal and professional development...and for contributions to social justice" (p. 21). This dimensional analysis reveals the nature of action research as being more than a research technique (method); rather it is an ethos—a common purpose or character that determines action (ethos, n.d.). The nature of action research is creating knowledge and applying it at the same time, merging theory and practice through reflection and reflexive practices.

To understand the essence of action research, it is important to review its origins and characteristics. This section provides a brief overview of the origins of action research and its processes, discusses *action research as an ethos* and outlines the influence of existentialism and wisdom perspectives as action research discourses.

History of Action Research

Because of the variation in action research activities, it is difficult to identify one concrete historical account of action research. If we consider that some of the philosophical origins of action research can be traced back to, for example, Habermas, Dewey, Marx, and Gadamer, it is easy to see why a specific line of history is difficult. However, Greenwood and Levin (2007) feel it is possible to map a general conceptual history and outline three genealogical strands: industrial democracy, the liberationist movement, and human inquiry.

The industrial democracy movement marked the beginning of research projects that were aimed at improving efficiencies in management and operations of organizations. These early projects were still influenced by Taylor's "scientific management" (Adelman, 1993) with inherent top-down-management approaches. Kurt Lewin's work in the 1930s, however, presented a different approach grounded in social change and democratic participation (Lewin, 1946). This social science research was considered "natural," where "researchers in a real-life context invited or forced participants to take part in an experimental activity" (Greenwood & Levin, 2007, p. 16). With a strong background in behavioral modification, Lewin outlined a three-stage process: breaking apart (unfreezing), changing, and re-forming (freezing) a structure.

Other projects that were significant in this industrial movement include the Tavistock Institute in the United Kingdom, the Swedish and Norwegian Industrial Democracy projects, and Levin's work at the University of California, Los Angeles. These projects were significant to furthering the conceptual understanding of action research and included three schemes: sociotechnical thinking, psychological job demands, and semiautonomous groups. Overall, the industrial democracy movement focused on improving participants' ability to control their own work environments and introduced a reflective, democratic process among participants and researchers (Greenwood & Levin, 2007).

During the liberationist movement, action research was employed to inequality, exploitation, and oppression, and was illustrated by an era of independence movements around the world. This movement against the inequalities of society formed the basis of Southern Participatory Action Research, Participatory Research, and Participatory Community Development (Greenwood & Levin, 2007). The significance of the liberationist movement in the history of action research is its emphasis on community and equalizing power relationships.

Human inquiry approaches to action research emerged on the scene in 1977 with the New Paradigm Research Group in London. "Shaping the 'humanness' in research" (Greenwood & Levin, 2007) was the central focus where the researcher becomes part of the research process. The historical significance of this approach to action research is its growing emphasis on personal and emotional elements of human inquiry and the engagement of the researcher as co-participant in the research process.

Action research in education primarily draws from the work of Lewin, followed by specific work with teacher-managed projects by Stephen Corey (Kemmis & McTaggart, 1988), and the British Humanities Curriculum Project lead by Lawrence Stenhouse and John Elliot (Adelman, 1993). In addition, the Ford Teaching Project, pioneered by Elliot and Adelman, focused on teachers using Enquiry learning (Adelman, 1993), and in Australia, Kemmis and McTaggart extended the work in the United Kingdom with an additional focus on Aboriginal education.

What Is Action Research?

According to Greenwood and Levin (2007), action research is social research comprised of a team that includes a professional researcher and members of a group, organization, or community. The major premise of action research is collaborative problem analysis and solving through a democratic and in-clusive process. Three elements together constitute action research—action, research, and participation—which aim to create knowledge for the purpose of social change. A key concept is that "action research democratizes research processes through the inclusion of the local stakeholders as co-researchers" (Greenwood & Levin, 2007, p. 3).

The general premise of action research is based on Lewin's approach in-volving a spiral of steps that include planning, action, observation, and eval-uation/reflection (Kemmis & McTaggart, 1988). Action research begins with an idea for improvement or change, then a group decides where to begin to make the change. This collective starting point allows group members to see where there are commonalities of perceived issues, forming the "thematic concern" they will focus on. This stage is the beginning of the reconnaissance stage of action research.

John Elliot (1991) criticized the simplistically straightforward nature of Lewin's original model and suggested that action research should also allow for the general idea to change. This evolving model includes ongoing analysis and fact-finding and only involves evaluation after there is awareness as to the extent to which action has occurred. Thus, Elliot (1991) describes a "spiral of cycles" (p. 70) that involves a basic cycle (identification of an idea, recon-naissance, planning, development of first action step, evaluation, revision of plan) and a spiral of additional steps (second action step, implementation, evaluation, revision of plan, develop third action step, etc.).

In the education context, action research is a form of applied research that educators can use to examine teaching and learning processes, problems at the individual, school, and/or district level, and professional growth (Alberta Teachers' Association, 2000). Action research in schools provides an oppor-tunity for educators to enhance their practice and skills, as well as gain con-nection to the world outside the walls of the classroom (Stringer, 2008, p. 2). Kemmis and McTaggart (1988) stress that action research provides a way for the school community to "live with the complexity of real experience while, at the same time, striving for concrete improvement" (p. 7).

Action Research as an Ethos

While many researchers and practitioners consider action research as a "methodology" with multiple steps, the nature of action research is not merely to apply these steps in a predetermined way to acquire knowledge about a

phenomenon. Noffke (2009) emphasizes that "action research is a set of commitments, rather than a set of techniques for research" (p. 21). Altrichter,
Kemmis, McTaggart and Zuber-Skerritt (2002) explain:

> Action research is about people reflecting upon and improving their own practice; by
> tightly inter-linking their reflection and action; and making their experiences public
> to other people concerned by and interested in the respective practice. (p. 128)

Action research is an ethos that is relational, reciprocal, participatory, and
emancipatory, and it seeks to democratize power relationships among participants and researchers (Herr & Anderson, 2005). The democratic process is
important in action research as it values multiple perspectives and expects dynamic participation and collaboration of stakeholders in a particular setting.

The uniqueness of action research is its ability to create knowledge and
apply knowledge at the same time. This "doing and thinking about it" approach is in contrast to bureaucratic research where the end product is ratio-
nally planned and measured. Interestingly, paying attention to the pathway
and conclusion essentially merges the theory/practice gap because epistemological and ontological concerns are considered together and "who one *is* becomes completely caught up in what one knows and does" (Sumara & Carson,
1997, p. xvii).

Having a theoretical understanding of wisdom traditions, existentialism,
action research, and *currere* perspectives provides the necessary base for a
more *complicated conversation* (Pinar, 1994) about curriculum and what happens when action research and *currere* flow together with wisdom. This will
provide a foundation for subsequent chapters where the inquiry journey begins and the notion of wisdom-guided inquiry is described in detail.

· 3 ·

LOCATING OURSELVES IN
CURRICULUM INQUIRY

"*Who* is doing the research is just as important as *what* research is being done and *how*."
— DAVID SMITH (2011B, P. 5)

Curriculum inquiry is the "focused investigation of a matter of public and/or private interest through asking questions; searching and (re)searching; paying attention/observing/ articulating; reading and writing; and dialogue" (Donald, 2011, p. 1). Smith (2011b) explains,

> It is the regrettable truth, however, that most educational research today is so narrowly defined as to reveal the multiples ways it has become disconnected from the historical, philosophical, economic and political roots of the world in which educational practices take place. (p. 1)

Thus, as researchers we must engage in curriculum inquiry "in a manner meaningful to our own interests, preoccupations, and musings" (Donald, 2011, p. 1), and engage *in* our research as situated participants *within* the inquiry. The situatedness of inquiry involves our own backgrounds and assumptions in relation to the collective other, and requires a disposition that questions and revisits our preconceived notions of our topic (Greene, 1973).

If curriculum is about the "journey of life" and "what the older generation choses to tell younger generations" (Grumet, 1980), then "what sorts of stories do we wish to tell the young?... How should curriculum conceptualize the past, address our present condition, and envision the future?" (Donald, 2011, p. 1). To address these questions, I believe researchers must begin their research by locating themselves within their projects. We must decide what stories we are going to tell and why we choose these stories in relation to what is being said and what is happening in our field. To open our eyes to the "power of the possible," to challenge our own assumptions, and interrogate the collective life history of our field, we must be willing to locate ourselves in our inquiry—temporally and spatially, as well as historically, politically, ethically, and philosophically. This also provides a more thorough understanding of the issues and background within the field of physical education that are significant to discussion about curriculum.

My own process of locating myself in curriculum inquiry (literally and metaphorically) involved an adaptation of the method of *currere* where the past (regressive) and imagining the future (progressive) is understood (analytic) for the self to be expanded, complicated, and mobilized (synthetical moment) (Pinar, 1994, 2004). This was not just an academic exercise; this part of the curriculum inquiry was/is deeply personal, embodied, and autobiographical. It reveals some of my past life experiences and visions for the future as a daughter, physical education teacher, athlete, coach, student, researcher, curriculum policy analyst, and curriculum consultant, and is shaped by my own struggles to maintain balance and wellness in my life. My stories are presented woven together with my re-entry into the present moment, attempting to illustrate my increased conceptual understandings and deeper knowledge with specific examples of connections within my field of study I made at the time (Pinar, 1994). Pinar (2004) explains, "the regressive-progressive-analytic-synthetic does not occur in discrete temporal or conceptual units, but simultaneously" (p. 131). Thus, some synthetical moments, "what occurs within and through the body [to] become a discernible whole, integrated in its meaningfulness," (p. 37) are found in this chapter (in italics), and you will find further synthetical moments throughout the book as you follow my journey to live a curriculum of wellness.

Place

From the time the Indian first set foot upon this continent, he centered his life in the natural world. He is deeply invested in the earth, committed to it both in his consciousness and in his instinct. The sense of place is paramount. Only in reference to the earth can he persist in his identity. (Momaday, 1994, as cited in Basso, 1996, p. 35)

*I grew up on a small farm in the Okanagan Valley. Our house was built in the middle
of the orchard and apple, plum, prune, pear, apricot and cherry trees surrounded
me. On the north side of our property was a shopping centre, on the south side there
was another orchard, to the east was the busy highway, and on the western slope was
a creek with dense shrubs, bushes, and mainly deciduous trees. The creek area was
a unique habitat for many living things, such as a family of herons, various species
of other birds, slugs, carp, snails, mice, wild cats, frogs, blackberries, Saskatoon
berries, chokecherry trees, cottonwoods, Oregon grape, poison ivy, and more. The
entire area was approximately 10 acres, eight of which were orchard and our family
dwelling.*

Places hold significance beyond being a patch of earth or stones. According
to Casey (1996),

> the lived body—the body living (in) a place is "the natural subject of perception."
> The experience of perceiving...requires a corporeal subject who lives in a place
> through perception.... Thus place integrates with the body as much as body with
> place. (p. 22)

Basso calls this dynamic *interanimation*—a relationship between people and
places that exist as interrelated and co-dependent phenomena (Bradley &
Mackinlay, 2007). Doerr (2004) believes "there is a wholeness to our lives
that can be found in a genuine relationship with place" (p. 22). Our family
farm, in its wholeness, provokes memories of knowing this place through my
senses and mind. It invokes a re-creation of the lessons learned associated
with the land and what it means to be a balanced, whole person in body,
mind, and spirit.

Mindfulness, Awareness and Stillness

*My ongoing relationship with trees began when I was four years old during the build-
ing of our new family home in the orchard. As a small child, being surrounded
by trees, all with their unique characteristics, was my way of life. I wandered up,
down, and between the rows when I played, and worked in the trees when doing
the many chores throughout the seasons. I had a favorite tree—a big, old, knotted
tree—that had a big trunk with a low fork that made it easy to climb. Planted by my
great grandfather, the tree was reaching the twilight years of his life cycle. He was a
wise friend and I used to sit in his branches and talk to him—he knew all my secrets,
hardships, and celebrations throughout my early childhood. It is not that the tree*

would literally speak to me; I just knew that every time I talked to him, he listened,
and somehow I knew everything would balance out. It was a sense, a feeling in my
being, a message of patience and calm.

The lowest "Y" of the tree provided a step for me to climb to his first main
branch, which was perfect for lying down. I would look up through his branches to
the bright blue sky and watch the birds and bugs traverse his branches and leaves. In
the late summer, I mostly just sat below the tree so not to disturb the apples. Although
it was not far from the busy highway, when I was in the tree, it was quiet, still. It was
a safe, happy place for me where I was able to feel the energy of the land, water, air,
and other living things around me.

John Welwood (1992) explains this pure childhood sense of wonder at
being alive as "wakeful presence." He believes that

> it is only in the stillness and simplicity of presence—when we are aware of what we
> are experiencing, when we are here with it as it unfolds—that we can really appreci-
> ate our life…and being alive on this earth. (p. xiv)

As a child playing in the trees, I was not concerned or distracted by what
was going on across the street or what I had to do later; I paid full attention
to the present moment. When we become distracted, we lose our ability to
be present and our minds begin to spin, taking us further away from balance
with the body and spirit. This fast-paced swirling is easy to achieve in our
materialistic world, as technology has increased our speed of communication,
cars, computers, and accessibility to television, phones and entertainment,
to such a level that we have very few gaps of time that are not filled. "When
we practice awareness instead of spinning out in thought, we 'find our seat':
We discover nowness, our most trustworthy ground and support" (Welwood,
1992, p. xxiii).

While there is some variation in the meaning of mindfulness, most descriptions refer to mindfulness as a conscious awareness of present action
(which includes stillness) in a nonjudgmental way. Roberts and Danoff-
Burg (2010) claim that mindfulness involves having awareness "that involves purposely focusing on the experiences of the present moment"
(p. 165). Francis and Lu (2009) describe mindfulness as "*mirror-thought* because mindfulness reflects or mirrors what is truly before us" (p. 24). Kabat-
Zinn (1994) refers to mindfulness "simply as the art of conscious living"
(p. 6) and explains how

it is simply a practical way to be more in touch with the fullness of your being through a systematic process of self-observation, self-inquiry, and mindful action.... The overall tenor of mindfulness practice is gentle, appreciative, and nurturing. Another way to think of it would be "heartfulness." (p. 6)

According to Markula (2004), in sport, physical education, and other physical activity disciplines, being mindful while performing movement activities involves proprioceptive awareness, focused breathing, proper body alignment and physical form, flow of intrinsic energy, and noncompetitive mental awareness. This view of mindfulness, however, is missing the philosophical dimensions that are important to healthy living. As Lu, Tito, and Kentel (2009) explain, "a physical education and health approach based on mindfulness... presents a holistic model of the human being according to which the body as object and body as subject are integrated" (p. 354). These authors also consider mindfulness as being the "basis of a subjective approach to the body that can bring added dimensions to physical education and lead to a holism that reflects more fully what it is to be human and that can lead to greater health" (p. 356).

Reciprocity

When you grow up on a farm, your life is organized according to the natural rhythms of the earth, as the trees' growing cycles do not follow the artificial fiscal and academic calendars we have imposed on our lives. The trees will tell you when it is time, so you must listen and watch. In the winter, the trees are "resting" and this is when we take the opportunity to prune their branches. It is best to prune before the warmth of the spring season, as the tree's circulatory system is dormant. A tree pruned during the late spring and summer will "bleed" and the shock of this can sometimes kill the tree.

Before the leaves and blossoms come out in the spring, we apply dormant-oil spray (lime-sulfur/oil spray) to smother wintering spores and fungus. Dormant spray is an organic defense against disease but it will damage leaves and fruit, so you must spray the trees before the buds open. In the spring, it is blossom season and it is time for our bee neighbors to visit and cross-pollinate the flowers. By June you begin to see the tiny apples forming from each pollinated flower.

As the apples grew on our farm, my dad would regularly walk throughout the orchard to inspect their progress. The trees would let him know when it was time to begin the process of thinning out the growth. Thinning not only helps the tree to carry the load

of the fruit on its limbs, but also ensures good development of colour, size, and shape of
the apples, and proper formation of flower buds for the following year. It is somewhat of
an art to thin apple trees in an effective and timely manner. I once asked my mom how
she did it and she said, "When you're up in the ladder amongst the leaves, branches,
and apples, somehow you just know. You hardly have to look—you just know the tree.
When you get down from the ladder, you step back and you can see what a branch can
handle. You just have to pay attention to what you're doing and enjoy it."

The fall was harvest season and again, the trees would be the ones to tell us
when to pick their fruit. The color, smell, taste, and texture of the apples, as well
as the weight of the fruit on the branches told us when it was time. It required daily
attentiveness and awareness of each block of trees because not all trees mature their
fruit at the same rate. We took great care to pick the apples, as we were respectful
of the trees' efforts to produce the nourishment that we were going to receive. Even
the apples that fall on the ground were picked up and made into juice or fruit leather.

The mutual respect that exists between the trees and the farmer is what
makes it all work. It was an unspoken understanding that we would take
care of the trees, and in return the trees would take care of us. This intimate
connection between the trees and our family is a viewpoint shared by many
Indigenous cultures around the world. Reciprocity reflects the belief that humans live interdependently with all forms of life, and our spiritual, emotional,
social, and mental health is dependent upon our harmonious relationship
with nature. Salmon (2000) explains how the traditions of the Raramuri,
who live in the eastern Sierra Madres of Mexico, "reveal the complexities of
the indigenous perceptions of self and culture intertwined in the web of life"
(p. 1328). The Raramuri believe that they came from the ears of corn following a great flood and destruction of the previous world. Thus, they prepare and
drink their corn beer, *batarik*, during ceremonies rituals, dances, and songs. It
is through these traditions that the Raramuri's connections to the Creator
become stronger, where "rain is assured and therefore, the life of the land and
the plants, animals, and people" (Salmon, 2000. p. 1328).

Being attuned to the natural rhythms of the Earth was very important
to maintain the reciprocal relationship with the land, trees, and other living
things in the orchard. This is also a significant part of the Blackfoot way of
life. A calendar date does not determine the start of the Sun Dance ceremony; the ripening of the Saskatoon berries does. This marks a time of great
thanksgiving, where many people come together and participate in sacred
ceremonies, including honoring the sun, as it is believed that all power comes

through the sun (Oakley, 2011). Another example of reciprocal relationships is evident in this Native American elder's explanation:

> The tree breathes what we exhale. When the tree exhales, we need what the tree exhales. So, we have a common destiny with the tree. We are all from the Earth and when the Earth—the water, the land, the atmosphere—is corrupted, then it will create its own reaction.... You should learn how to plant something, that's the first connection. You should treat all things as spirit; realize that we are all one family. (Westerman, 2008)

This notion of reciprocation is an example of a way of living life, a mindful way of being *in* the world.

From Disconnectedness to "Wide-Awakeness"

I began my teaching career in Kamloops, British Columbia, the year of the 1993 Canada Summer Games. At the time, I was the head coach for the city track-and-field club and was asked to be the meet director for athletics at the games. Along with my years as a high-performance athlete and physical education teacher training, this was a significant event in my mind-body disconnect. There was little time or space for me to stop and pay attention to anything but preparing for the games and the new school year. During the games, they brought an RV on site for me to sleep in, as co-ordinating 400 volunteers, 150 officials, 600 athletes and coaches, and juggling the media, contractors, and general manager did not allow me time to go home to sleep. Ten days after the closing ceremonies, I began my first year teaching and coaching. My life was focused on performance, end-goals, efficiencies, winning, effective techniques, measurement, and scheduling. My teaching practices relied heavily on the sport model with objective performance dominating my assessment practices. I was coaching senior girls' volleyball four nights a week and going to tournaments on the weekends. My 16-hour days did not include time for myself. I was living in an area of Kamloops surrounded by buildings, traffic, and pavement, driving 60 minutes to work morning and night. I never stopped to reflect on what I was doing; I was just surviving. I did not have any connection to nature, other than the grass in the middle of the track, nor did I have any connection with my own spirit. Essentially, my body and mind were separate; it was like I was living outside of my own body.

With all the "noise" and "spinning" in my life at this time, I was not grounded or present in body, mind, heart, and spirit (Welwood, 1992). I had turned my back on what was so innately part of my life as a child, thus I was out of touch with life in and around me. As a coach, there was a distinct sub-ject–object and body–mind dichotomy. Unknowingly, we trained athletes to look at the body as an object. The athlete body was for a purpose—the pursuit of the win, that Gold Medal. We trained in snow, sleet, and rain to gain an advantage, to become more efficient and effective. We analyzed body angles, forces, take-offs, and landings, and we read the latest research on new techniques. Students trained through minor injuries, competed with taped-up ankles, applied ice between races—whatever was needed to keep going. It is no surprise that this was my experience too as an athlete when I was a teenager.

My physical education program reflected a traditional sport approach where we focused primarily on product not process. It was mostly about how many serves went in the target, balls in the hoop, shots in the net—always pushing students to do more, to be better. It was an environment preoccu-pied with posted standards and students were "put on stage" in comparison to their classmates. At the time, I did not realize that this objective, empirical approach to physical education is somewhat counterproductive to the goal of physical education—to gain the knowledge, skills, and attitude to be healthy and active for life. The objective approach often leads to a "more is better" ap-proach and excludes other dimensions that foster better holistic health (e.g., social, emotional, spiritual health) (Lu, Tito, & Kentel, 2009).

Maxine Greene (1973) challenges us "to do philosophy" (p. 7), but in the demanding day-to-day business of the school, teachers conduct their lessons with little thought about the underlying principles that guide what they think, how they teach, and why they do what they do (Greene, 1984b). A teacher must therefore probe and ask questions to try to understand what impinges on her daily teaching practice and be able to "bracket out" presuppositions that may limit her vision to one dimension. While difficult for beginning teachers, doing philosophy means being "wide-awake" to the multiplicity of realities that consti-tute the life-world of a teacher (Greene, 1978). Being wide-awake also includes nurturing mindfulness and presence. It was time for me to become wide-awake.

Stranger in a New Land

After three years teaching, I began graduate work in Victoria, British Columbia, and began to question the focus of physical education curriculum. My research with female students about their experiences in physical education was eye-opening and forced me to examine my own teaching practice. Participants expressed their dislike for physical education and did not see the relevance of playing basketball, floor hockey, volleyball, and soccer (for the twelfth year in a row) to their lives outside of the school environment. They wanted to "have fun," participate, and learn about things that would be possible for them to do on their own. I began to understand that physical education needed to be more than learning the technical skills to play traditional sports.

It was apparent to me that I was too focused on just one element of the child, the physical. Our teacher education program focused on teaching efficiency, technical skill progressions, and rules of games. While the physical is an important aspect of being healthy, the whole child is more than one dimension. I realized that our industrial model of education had forced us into fragmented practices where we separate children's bodies and minds into compartments. The whole child was broken into bits and pieces to be addressed in different classrooms throughout the school. There was (and is) little connection between the subject areas in junior/senior high school and even less connection to the community, land, or world. Unfortunately, at that point, I was still looking at physical education as an outsider, as an interesting topic to be studied. In my experience I never disliked participating in physical activities. It was not until I was nearing the end of my master's degree that a significant event forced me to see things in a different way.

I was teaching part-time when I was involved in an accident where I collided with a student during physical education class. I landed on the base of my neck and hit my head on the frozen ground with significant force. The ensuing months and years proved to be some of the most challenging of my life. The post-concussive symptoms made it impossible for me to teach, and I took medical leave to participate in a full-time rehabilitation program. My short- and long-term memory was impacted, as were my motor skills. I was easily confused and frustrated, and managing simple household tasks had to be relearned. I worked with physical and occupational therapists who assisted me with re-establishing neural-muscular pathways and learning new strategies for staying organized. Progress was slow and it became apparent that my future physical education teaching days were in doubt.

As my difficulties with processing information, problem solving, and abstract thinking improved, I began to think about myself as a teacher. The frustrating experiences in my rehabilitation program when I was unable to perform simple motor-skill tasks provided me with a new lens. The recovery from the accident allowed me to understand that my teaching had been focused on performing the correct skill sequences (psychomotor), knowing the rules and technique cues (cognitive), and demonstrating effort (affective). My students were forced to fit into this traditional approach. I assumed the students would get satisfaction and enjoyment from improving and/or *excelling at the skills, which would then lead to being more successful when playing. This had been my experience in junior/senior high school and what I learned in my teacher education program.*

My time in rehabilitation taught me something new, and I began to understand how demoralizing it is to be asked to perform a movement activity that I was incapable of doing regardless of how much effort I put into it. Fortunately, I had therapists who adjusted my program to meet my needs and found activities and strategies I could be successful at. Just saying "good effort" every session did not motivate me when I hated the fact that I could not complete the tasks. This experience connected to my physical education classes because we evaluated heavily on "effort and participation." I started to realize what my students' lived experiences were like in my physical education classes.

With the lingering symptoms of my injury as a reminder, I knew that if I wanted to continue in this profession, I would have to change my philosophy of teaching physical education. I would have to start finding new ways to engage my students and make physical education class more meaningful for them.

Greene (1973) calls for teachers to "take a stranger's vantage point on everyday reality...to look inquiringly and wonderingly on the world in which one lives" (p. 267). The stranger is like someone who has returned home from a long trip. She sees her environment in a way she has never seen before. Everything that was familiar before now seems foreign. She is looking through new lenses and to make things meaningful again "(s)he must interpret and reorder what (s)he sees in the light of [her] changed experience" (p. 268). My head injury and rehabilitation was a long trip, and it changed me. I was a stranger in a land I did not recognize. To understand how to get around in this new land, I had to ask for directions (from mentors who were teaching with a holistic perspective) and needed a new map (a new curriculum). Greene's (1971) advice in this situation is:

> He himself may recognize that he will have to come to understand the signs on the map if he is to make use of it. Certainly he will have to decipher the relationship between those signs and "real objects in the city." But his initial concern will be conditioned by the "objects" he wants to bring into visibility, by the landmarks he needs to identify if he is to proceed on his way. (p. 140)

As *physical education teacher as stranger,* I began to question my own assumptions and make myself dissonant to the positivist approach that I now knew students were already questioning. As stranger, I began to hear the voices of my inactive, disengaged students, and their reasons for disliking physical education—boredom, irrelevance to their lives, negative peer interactions, a lack of connection to the curriculum (both curriculum-as-lived and curriculum-as-plan), and perceived lack of value of physical education (Gibbons, Wharf-Higgins, Gaul, & VanGyn, 1999; Humbert, 2006; Hunter, 2006; Kilborn, 1999).

Taking Care of Self and Other

I could no longer ignore the voices of students who said traditional, sport-based physical education was not meeting their needs. I searched for a more holistic approach where students had choice, understood how to take care of their physical selves, learned how to help each other, accepted each other's differences, and in the process, enjoyed participating in a class with a variety of physical activities. One of my units in Physical Education 9/10 was field lacrosse, where several of my students who played community lacrosse led the majority of instruction and activities (with my guidance). It was brilliant, as the confidence they had and brought out in others built throughout the two weeks. My students were becoming far more engaged than ever before. They began to feel empowered and to ask which activity they could lead next.

Another element I thought was missing in senior physical education classes was social responsibility. I asked my grade 11/12 students to watch our neighboring elementary school's recess and notice what was missing. They clearly observed that very few children were "playing." We discussed what they thought were the reasons for this and came to the conclusion that the games that used to get passed down from generation to generation had been lost. We then decided to organize a program where my Physical Education 11/12 students were responsible for learning, planning, and teaching a playground game to a class at the elementary school. It was an incredible learning experience for both sets of students, and later we began to see more students playing outside during lunch and recess. The best part is that the elementary students were playing the games that my students had taught them.

Greene (1988) believes that empowerment and freedom involves praxis and explains, "it is important to hold in mind…that the person—that center of choice—develops in his/her fullness to the degree he/she is a member of a live community" (p. 43). Transcendence occurs when we "wake up" and move out and beyond to change the world.

There is a moderate amount of research in the health and physical education field that relates to personal and social responsibility. Hellison's (2011)
work on teaching personal and social responsibility in physical activity focuses on "students taking more responsibility for their own development and
wellbeing and for supporting the wellbeing of others" (p. 6) through awareness. A social critical perspective accepts that all knowledge is value laden.
Researchers try to make explicit the assumptions about physical education, including a commitment to social justice, equity, inclusivity, and social change
(Macdonald et al., 2002). Socially critical research in physical education
emerged in the 1980s when researchers began to direct their inquiries toward
equality, social justice, and emancipation, and question traditional views of
physical education research and practice. These critiques of the technical
model of physical education offer alternative approaches to overcome positivistic limitations, encourage personal and social responsibility among students,
and empower teachers to be social change agents (Devis-Devis, 2006).

Fernandez-Balboa (1997) has considered a social-critical pedagogical approach to physical education that involves empowerment, democracy, and
student-centered practices. This is an environment where

> students are encouraged to take leadership and ownership in the learning process;
> jointly pose questions and problems; determine (or at least critique and suggest) the
> course content; and apply knowledge to personal, social and political contexts. Here
> learning becomes humanizing and emancipatory." (p. 134)

Wellness

*My move to Alberta Education introduced me to a way to think about my field in a
different way. Students should be learning how to take care of themselves and others,
where they are focused on the balance of all dimensions of wellness—physically,
emotionally, spiritually, and mentally. Hence, the notion of introducing wellness
education in the K–12 education system was now firmly planted in my mind. The
question was, however, what does wellness mean? The attempt to answer this question was a massive undertaking that took over two years and challenged my own personal health and wellness. However, the result was a new "Framework for Wellness
Education in Alberta."*

Wellness education presents a conceptual shift that reflects a holistic approach across all curricula, and combines previously separated health-related

and physical education programs of study. This type of educational change requires a vision that communicates, motivates, and inspires school communities to move towards improving student health and wellness. Recommendations from a wellness curricula literature review conducted in 2007 emphasized the importance of developing a comprehensive description of wellness before continuing with program development (Alberta Education, 2008). Thus, a wellness definition for the province was created so education stakeholders would have a common understanding of what wellness means in the context of the education system. Multiple stakeholders, including parents; students; teachers; administrators; community members; and First Nations, Métis, Inuit, and Francophone groups designed an overall definition of wellness and descriptions of each dimension of wellness—emotional, intellectual, physical, social, and spiritual (Table 1).

Table 1. *Definitions of the dimensions of wellness.*

Emotional wellness is acknowledging, understanding, managing, and expressing thoughts and feelings in a constructive manner.

Intellectual wellness is the development and the critical and creative use of the mind to its fullest potential.

Physical wellness is the ability, motivation, and confidence to move effectively and efficiently in a variety of situations, and the healthy growth, development, nutrition, and care of the body.

Social wellness is relating positively to others and is influenced by many factors, including how individuals communicate, establish and maintain relationships, and are treated by others and interpret that treatment.

Spiritual wellness is an understanding of one's own values and beliefs, leading to a sense of meaning or purpose and a relationship to the community.

(Alberta Education, 2009, p. 3)

Walking Away...A Step Closer to Wellness?

I was excited about the approval of the framework and anxious to start putting it into action. We had collected many innovative and exciting ideas as we went around the province. I could see such great potential. We had momentum and many of the participants who contributed to the framework were eager to get started. In a short period of time, however, it became clear that the Ministry was supportive of the concept, but not necessarily supportive of taking action. I did what I could to move the project forward, but it seemed that the notion of wellness education was destined to remain just words on paper.

I was finishing my contract with Alberta Education and wondered if there was any way that this work could be continued "on the outside." Personally and professionally I had grown so much and wanted to continue the progress I had made. So, I decided to apply to graduate studies, hoping to continue to pursue my shift in philosophy towards a more holistic approach. I arrived at the University of Alberta with the knowledge I gained from co-developing the Wellness Education Framework with no idea how I would navigate this new environment that did not have anyone doing research in wellness education. Admittedly, I immediately compromised and labeled my research interest as "the role of health and physical education curriculum in a health promoting schools approach."

My awareness of the readiness of my own field to shift to "wellness" was part of my reason for adjusting my research inquiry. In addition, there has been some success in implementing a health promoting schools model in schools in Alberta (APPLE Schools, 2013; Ever Active Schools, n.d.), and this approach I felt was philosophically similar to the idea of wellness. The origins of the concept of health promotion came from a similar place as the need for wellness.

The concept of health promotion in schools originated from public health professionals' concern that health education programs had become too individualistic and placed the responsibility for health solely on the individual, absolving society and government of all obligations to address health. A broader perspective, health promotion, is considered a proactive strategy that moves away from the disease-oriented medical approach. It emphasizes a more empowering, holistic model that involves the development of individual's skills and self-determination, but also the utilization of social and personal resources to maintain a state of wellbeing (McCuaig, 2006; Simovska, 2004).

Predictably, the schools became a major focus for health-promotion advocates, as it was recognized that the "interaction between schools and young people, and the overall experience of attending school, provides unique opportunities for health promotion which can be sustained and reinforced over time" (National Health and Medical Research Council, 1996, as cited in McCuaig, 2006, p. 60). This opportunity materialized in the World Health Organization's health promoting schools approach as an international framework where school communities work together to plan and facilitate health promoting school programs.

A health promoting schools approach is commonly defined as a "whole-school approach to enhancing both the health and educational outcomes of children and adolescents through learning and teaching experiences initiated in the schools" (International Union for Health Promotion and Education [IUHPE], 2010, p. 5). Health promoting schools (referred to as comprehensive school health in Canada) involves linking learning beyond the formal curriculum to the home, school, and community. Such an approach incorporates four interrelated components: healthy school policies, physical and social environments, teaching and learning, and partnerships and services (Joint Consortium for School Health, n.d.).

As part of the health promoting schools model, the World Health Organization (WHO) also recommends curriculum perspectives that focus on individual health skills and action competencies. Emphasis is on the need to move from a topics approach to a holistic approach where students are able to consider issues in the "reality of the social and environmental contexts of their lives" (IUHPE, 2010, p. 4). This approach can be further defined as:

> both the formal and informal curriculum and associated activities, where students gain age-related knowledge, understandings, skills and experiences, which enable them to build competencies in taking action to improve the health and wellbeing of themselves and others in their community and that enhances their learning outcomes. (IUHPE, 2010, p. 3)

Wisdom and Wellness

My personal inquiry took me in many different directions, but one thing I kept coming back to is my experiences with the First Nations, Métis, and Inuit Elders during my time at the Ministry of Education. During the process of developing the framework, I was asked to take all the stories and descriptions from hundreds of participants and filter them down to five or six. When we took the framework document back to the Elders, they were disappointed. Through stories and some debate, they told us that we did not capture the essence of wellness as they know it. This I understand, as I know what was on the "cutting-room floor" and I personally heard the wisdom that was in each of those rooms across the province. I now know what the elders were saying—wellness is more than a definition; it is a way of "being" in this world, how we live our lives, how we connect to others and the Earth. So recently, when considering my work in curriculum and health promoting schools, I have been thinking, "where are the trees?" I have not read anything in the health promoting

schools research that captures the idea of the reciprocal relationship between people
and the sacred processes of the Earth.

The health promoting schools approach considers the social and physical environments in the schools, as well as the social and emotional dimension of students, but little reference is made to basic connectivity humans have to the rhythms of nature. While the health promoting schools approach invites students, teachers, and schools to connect learning activities beyond the school and to consider the social and environmental context of students' lives, it is very policy driven with promises to solve the ills of society and prepare students for the world "out there" (the global competitive market)—a future that exists outside themselves. I believe what is missing from this approach is a wisdom perspective.

Whether we consider Buddhism, Confucianism, Christianity, Taoism, Hinduism, or Indigenous traditions, the common thread among all wisdom traditions is the notion that "life has a *Way* to it, a Way to live that is compatible with, or co-extensive with the very manner of Life's unfolding" (Smith, 2008a, p. 2). The idea that we have fragmented everything in the school system, including health and wellness, speaks to how we have broken the fundamental unity of the world that wisdom traditions support. Smith (2011a) believes we must begin a discussion about

> wisdom and the requirements of healthy living and human wellbeing, since it is a mark of all wisdom traditions that the world inheres in a fundamental unity that cannot be broken except artificially as an act of human will. Human wellbeing depends on a unity between word and act, between self and other, and between the human and natural worlds, and between life and death. (p. 171)

The challenge when considering wisdom-guided curriculum is to avoid the commodification that currently dominates many of the wisdom tradition practices that have been adopted in Western culture. One only has to do a simple online search to understand how practices such as meditation and yoga have become some of the most marketed "products" with clothing, self-help books, DVDs, and music promising instant health and wellbeing. This includes educational resources as well. Smith (2011a) explains,

> practic[ing] meditation so as a teacher you may more calmly orchestrate the pedagogical and curricular necessities of daily life…is exactly wrong, since it merely sponsors and nurtures the kind of happy dissociation, or cultural schizophrenia that is at the heart of the problem. (p. 172)

This does not mean we abandon wisdom traditions in schools altogether; we need to be sure we understand what wisdom means in health- and wellness-related curriculum. Wisdom traditions

> regard health as intrinsic to our nature, and thus already fully present within us. The source of health is…our wakeful awareness, clarity, vitality and caring. Tuning into this intelligence at work in us can guide us toward living in a healthy way. (Welwood, 1992, p. 155)

Thus, there is value in meditative practice within a school program as a way to help students recover the "unity of their being…. Distractedness, inability to focus and concentrate… increasingly these qualities have come to define the lives of young people, which the wisdom curriculum may serve to heal" (Smith, 2011a, p. 175).

Location of Inquiry

The location of this inquiry is both temporal and spatial, thus the preceding weave of my actual events and times of my life story that were significant to my inquiry, and the relationships with various people, places, and living things. As mentioned previously, my journey to my current location has been via an adaptation of the method of *currere*. As Pinar further explains,

> This autobiographical method asks us to slow down, to remember even re-enter the past, and to meditatively imagine the future. Then, slowly and in one's own terms, one analyzes one's experience of the past and the fantasies of the future in order to understand more fully, with more complexity and subtlety, one's submergence in the present.

I am now situated in a position where I can see the potential for a curriculum of wellness, a holistic approach, and wisdom traditions within my field. However, I have yet to come to terms with how this will emerge within the positivistic nature of physical education, as well as within our fragmented education system. My hope is that this inquiry will provide a way to begin the conversation about our collective location in our field and consider the possibilities that "running the course" and a curriculum of wellness may offer.

I just came back from a run in the Edmonton river valley. The sun was brilliant, a sliver of moon was out, the sky was beyond blue, and the wind was cool but gentle.

As I passed through the trees, I noticed some birds building a nest—their songs were beautiful as they hurried to bring new twigs and materials to their new home. I could hear in the distance a big commotion and as I neared the river, I saw what it was. The ice had now broken up and pieces of every different size and shape were flowing by. I stopped to watch the festivities, as the young birds challenged each other to land on a moving piece of ice. It seemed that they all laughed when one of them missed and had to make a water landing. I looked around and it appeared that everyone/thing was in on the event—the riverbank, trees, and the older birds joined me as spectators to cheer the young birds on. It was as if this were an annual event. It probably is.

I continued my run, listening to the rhythm of my breath with every three or four steps and the beating of my heart in my ears. Two of the biggest geese I have ever seen were a few feet from the trail, rummaging whatever food they could find. The larger of the two looked up as I came near, as if to say hello, and continued to stare at me until I rounded the next bend in the trail. As I turned from gazing behind me, I nearly stepped on a little chipmunk as he scurried across the path and under the fence. He was in a hurry—no time to socialize, I guess.

I finish my run and sit in stillness under a tree and suddenly I am back home in the orchard.

This is my location right now. I am among the creatures of the Earth, the wind, sun, moon, water, riverbank, trees, leaves, birds, and so on. It is a time and place for awareness, stillness, and re-connecting. It is a time to sit with my inquiry and let the trees and other living things speak to me. This is a "way of life" that extends into my inquiry process—it is now whole. This "way" will help me and others get to a place of wellness where we are able to sit in, below, and around the trees, and be completely in sync with the rhythms of the tree and his surroundings. I can see and hear the tree. There is *a Way* to wellness. We just have to breathe, pay attention, feel, and listen to the wisdom that naturally exists in and around us.

· 4 ·

WISDOM-GUIDED INQUIRY

A MINDFUL JOURNEY

Sitting still or lying still, in any moment we can reconnect with our body, tran-
scend the body, merge with the breath, with the universe, experience ourselves
as whole and folded into larger and larger wholes. A taste of interconnectedness
brings deep knowledge of belonging, a sense of being an intimate part of things, a
sense of being at home wherever we are. We may taste and wonder at an ancient
timelessness beyond birth and death, and simultaneously experience the fleet-
ing brevity of this life as we pass through it, the impermanence of our ties to our
body, to this moment to each other. Knowing our wholeness directly in the meditation practice, we may find ourselves coming to terms with things as they are, a
deepening of understanding and compassion, a lessening of anguish and despair.
— JON KABAT-ZINN (1994, P. 226)

The term "inquiry" comes from the 13th-century Old French term *enquerre*,
meaning "to ask about" (inquire, n.d.). "To ask about" how someone teaches
must intimately involve the teacher in the process, consider the complexities
of practitioner research in a school setting and carefully consider the situatedness of the teacher. In other words, the way you choose to conduct research
determines the type and depth of knowledge about a question. If you look
beyond conventional empirical understandings of the term "methodology,"
and consider method in the broader ecological sense, originating from the
Greek (early 15th century) *methodos*, meaning "a way of teaching or going,"

using theoretical resources helps inform *how* you conduct your research and your analysis. In this case, inherent in the question we were asking about was a theoretical perspective that also guided "methodology."

In this chapter rather than merely providing a descriptive account, I will attempt to give the reader a sense, a feeling, an aesthetic understanding of the journey that Kim and I traveled on this wisdom-guided inquiry. I will first explain what we mean by wisdom-guided inquiry and our struggles during this process and "walk (run) you around" the actual journey highlighting the *currere* process, our way of living as co-researchers, and my reflections as an observer and participant over the course of the high school semester.

A Way of Being Co-Researchers

The teaching situation is filled with many different encounters and experiences that connect us to certain historical, political, cultural, and economic conditions, and we must research in *a way* that allows us to respond mindfully and pedagogically (Smith, 2013). This means you must pay attention to the way things really are. If you are presently aware as a researcher, you can see, hear, feel, sense, and experience the pedagogical moments as they are. This is the path, *the way*, of inquiry, of living in "research" that Kim and I traveled as co-researchers and what we refer to as a wisdom-guided mode of inquiry.

When we began our journey together, we were both somewhat uncertain about where it would all lead. Kim was nervous and commented that there is a level of vulnerability involved when someone watches you teach. But she explained,

> I think that is good for me and good for the class. I've always said it's not about me; it's about the students. If it was only about me and being the perfect teacher, I wouldn't take any advice—I wouldn't talk to anybody about this. So I don't mind putting myself out there.

She was open to sharing and learning. I was nervous, which meant I had to "let go" of my positivistic notions of research. Understanding that our question comes from a position of practice and being, I had to have faith that I was going to be informed and trust that in each moment there was something to be learned—as long as I paid attention and remained open-minded.

Common to wisdom traditions is the practice of being open and sharing. For example, openness means to see things the way they truly are in a given situation (Aristotle), with a consciousness that unifies Self and Other

(Buddhism, Hinduism), stillness (Christianity, Taoism, Hebrew) without distraction so that we are able to listen and feel more fully. The unification of Self and Other, *prajna* in Hinduism, allows one to be able to share of themselves freely, selflessly (Smith, 2013). Cree Elders believe that sharing is a natural way to build relationships, and when we share sacred knowledge, values, and life experience, we learn how to live well together (Hart, 1999).

To be able to pay attention to the present moment, one must participate fully in the world, in this case, the class. This is a mindful way of being where we learn how to live more deeply in the world—body, mind, and spirit. When you practice mindfulness in a research environment, you become aware of things that otherwise may go unnoticed as mindfulness brings together the emotional, spiritual, physical, and mental aspects of humanness. The mindful inquirer is "in touch in the present time" (*Tiep Hien*, Buddhism), what Thich Nhat Hanh (1987) calls "interbeing," which requires the use of all the senses, a connection at the spiritual level and promotes the oneness of the researcher with the researched (Bai, 2001).

To achieve mindfulness requires meditative practice, which "facilitates clearing the discursive mind" (Cohen & Bai, 2007, p. 6). A story from the Zen tradition:

空 A Cup of Tea

Nan-in, a Japanese master during the Meiji era (1868–1912), received a university professor who came to inquire about Zen.

Nan-in served tea. He poured his visitor's cup full, and then kept on pouring.

The professor watched the overflow until he no longer could restrain himself. "It is overfull. No more will go in!"

"Like this cup," Nan-in said, "you are full of your own opinions and speculations. How can I show you Zen unless you first empty your cup?" (Senzaki & Reps, 1957, p. 19).

The Chinese character 空 means empty, hollow.... Who comes to inquire? A professor, a learned man full of knowledge! What could be better? A professor comes to learn, *but*—and it's a very big but—the master sees that the professor is so filled with pre-conceived and pre-digested ideas that there is no room for fresh seeing of *what is*. (Cohen & Bai, 2007, p. 6)

As alluded to by the Zen master above, one must empty the mind to be able to see what is truly there. If we do not have awareness of when we hold onto all the past ideas, knowledge, concepts, and experiences, it is difficult to see anew. Thus, the autobiographical method of *currere* was an important activity because *currere* can guide us to a greater ontological understanding of the collective way of being by first understanding the self and the self in relation to the collective, in each regressive-progressive present moment. *Currere* "employs the past to reveal the present assumptions and future intention" (Pinar & Grumet, 1976, p. 73). This process is like an emptying because it allows us to name our dilemmas, "let go" of our attachments, and be open to new ideas. Being able to trace the roots of our understandings and seeing what is actually in front of us requires what Smith (2011a) terms as *meditative sensibility*. This has nothing to do with the commodified culture of meditation that is prevalent in the West where trendy studios offer step-by-step classes and market their books, clothing, and products. It is also not an "escape" from reality or a relaxation technique that will solve the ills of society—meditation sensibility allows us to see and name the issues and problems that swirl in our minds, consume our energy, and get us caught in what Beck (1993) refers to as clogged-up whirlpools and stagnant waters. Kumar (2013) describes meditation from Krishnamurti's view as a "kind of awareness [that] gives rise to an understanding or perception into the nature of things as they are without any distortion due to one's past experiences, memories and images" (p. 90).

While there was a structure to *currere* in the form of guiding questions that upon inspection seem to have a specific temporal expectation each week, in reality writing in this way fosters moments of regression and progression in the present to help us better understand what is truly at work in front of us. It frees you from mindless action and reveals possible meaning that we may not have been able to see otherwise. For myself, it was like multidimensional pinball pathways that were in constant motion simultaneously bouncing from the past-present-future to redefine the present moment. Noticing, observing, and discussing past events and experiences, or visioning the future, helps us interpret their significance for the present condition. Fowler (2006) understands this as revealing the curriculum of difficulty in teaching, working toward "rethink[ing] and rewrit[ing] the educational narrative" (p. 151). My co-researcher Kim also felt that it helped her name some problems, which aided in her ability to accept them and understand how they impacted her way of being. She joked about how therapeutic it was to reveal the relationship between past events and the present moment, and be able to "re-write" how she views the present moment while connecting it to her future vision. She commented how important understanding these relationships between the past-present-future were for her own health and wellness. *It starts with the self.*

Meditative practice was vital for me throughout the semester. Kim's scheduling of yoga on Mondays was not only an important factor for guiding students, but it established a way of starting the week that allowed both of us to "empty our cups." This extended into my own regular practice even on non-yoga days. Before I began observing/participating, I would spend at least five to ten minutes meditating, being still. Meditation can take place in many different forms and some may have a stereotypical image of a yoga master in a trance-like state, but really what it is about is silence and finding stillness in our mind. My meditative practice before entering the classroom took place in a variety of ways: sitting in my truck in the parking lot, going for a walk on the field, lying under a tree, or sitting/lying in the studio.

During our one-on-one conversations, Kim and I started each session with a moment where we just stopped, were silent, took a few deep breaths, and focused on each other in the room. It was as though the chaos, noise, and pressures outside the classroom door just faded. It allowed us to truly listen with our full attention given to each other "without the interference from the constant movement of thought" (Kumar, 2013, p. 91). In essence, there was no "division between the listener and the speaker…they become part of the whole where two things—the origination of the sound and the act of listening—are happening simultaneously" (p. 91). There was a feeling of calm that was present in our discussions, underscored by compassion, generosity, kindness, and respect. There was an energy and connection that was present for us to accept and foster a level of awareness of the pedagogical situation that I do not think would have been possible otherwise.

This connection between co-researchers is essential and akin to what is referred to as the *ethos* of action research. As previously described, *action research as an ethos* emphasizes that there is a moral disposition to the research process that guides action, where we simultaneously think, live, and act reflectively and reflexively. This goes beyond participation in a democratic process as you are *living* in the co-researcher relationship, and the experience of maintaining this collaborative relationship requires a nondualistic way of being. Nondualistic practice encourages letting go and allows us to see our attachment to specific views, opinions, and ideas. It encourages acceptance of being prepared to live in a space that accepts both the objective world and subjective experience as we need both to fully understand the nature of a phenomenon. Poonamallee (2009) explains this as a holistic philosophy that includes objective and subjective dimensions of reality in a noncontrary relationship. Knowledge and knowing is the tension, the struggle to live and understand in an objective epistemological *and* subjective ontological way, where each is constantly informing the other. It is particularly difficult to negotiate this relationship when you consider the traditional ways of knowing that are so deeply entrenched in our school system, and notably physical education, that value the mind over and separate from the body and spirit. As such, there is a resistance to knowing through both subjective and objective realities that sets up this either-or, "curriculum-as-planned *versus* curriculum-as-lived," or "is-is not" trap and inevitably extinguishes the possibility of multiple perspectives. It also sets up a rush to judgment, "the" solution, a focused quest for "an answer"—something prevalent in a field that is very focused on performance and end-product. There is a certain faith required in this kind of practice and a tolerance of waiting.

As co-researchers, Kim and I consciously had to resist our tendency to want to have the answer to the inquiry question NOW! We frequently identified and named this struggle for each other with the constant reminder to have patience and return to our breath so that we could notice the pedagogical moments and be able to mindfully discuss their significance. We also had to remind ourselves that the ongoing, active, dialogical, dialectical experience among the students, the political, historical, social situation, and ourselves is where we would learn. This was not a static moment in time, it was a journey—it was constantly evolving and we had to learn how to live in it, as individuals and together. It was within this unmapped journey that we gained knowledge.

Those engaged in action research recognize that the nature of the collaborative relationship sets up tensions that when carefully considered can impact the co-generative synchronic nature of knowledge creation and application. As this inquiry process was informed by action research, there are similar tensions, or what we referred to as struggles, at work. With the connection of body-mind-spirit, the spiritual experience involves the naming, acceptance, and living with/in the struggles of the inquiry and human condition. There is much to be learned in how we respond to these struggles and use the principles of balance/harmony to return to the heart so that we may see and listen at a deeper level.

There were issues of power relations that were present throughout the semester that are a part of the collaborative process and the political/social context of an educational setting. These power relations are rooted in the positionality of co-researchers, hierarchical structures within the school, dominant discourses within the physical education department, and perceived perception of teacher autonomy (Herr & Anderson, 2005). For example, the impact that my presence as a researcher in the classroom would have on Kim's students was something we discussed in our first meeting. Our concern was how it may affect Kim's relationship with students if they were only being observed or thought we were co-teaching the course. We discussed many considerations including: students may perceive that my position as university researcher meant I had "more knowledge" than Kim about holistic health, students would feel uncomfortable being "watched" from the sidelines and thereby feel self-conscious about participating in class, and having two adult "teachers" in the room could be intimidating and negatively affect Kim's ability to make connections with her students. We had to be aware that all of these scenarios could not only impact our ability to co-construct meaning related to our inquiry question but also have significant consequences to her students' experience in the overall course. This dialogue was not only an important piece to establishing a cooperative, collaborative relationship but also demonstrates a key principle of all wisdom traditions: the centrality of interconnectedness.

Many Indigenous cultures use the concept of the circle to represent that all living things are connected and "each is affected as much as any part of the circle is affected" (Pewewardy, 1999, p. 31). Understanding this reciprocity clearly highlights another way of being a researcher that is necessary for balancing power relationships, and a key principle of mindfulness—kind, compassionate living. Winter (2003) explains how kindness and compassion must start with "positive feelings of 'wishing well'" towards the self, then progressively to others (friends, acquaintances, and those who may be unfriendly).

This kind compassionate living comes into view with Kim's struggle and awareness of the other power relationships within the school setting. It is important to understand that by naming these power dynamics at play, she can subsequently through mindful practice let them go and in doing so, view them as pedagogical encounters. Kim's regressive accounts in the *currere* process are evident in how she has come to find balance with the social, political, historical, cultural situations within her school. The empathy and compassion that underlies her words and actions allows her to avoid getting entangled in the competitive, "higher-faster-stronger" discourse that runs through the hallways of our schools and feeds the growing systemic addiction to material gain and neglect of the spiritual dimension among our youth. Through wishing positive energy towards others, expressing joyful empathy in others' accomplishments, and a general understanding of the challenges and possibilities of human nature (Winter, 2003), Kim is able to *be* a teacher in a way that is inherently value laden and holistic.

We are not suggesting that this mindful practice was perfect, hence the term "practice." For example, one of Kim's struggles was what Aoki (as cited in Pinar & Irwin, 2005) refers to as dwelling in the tension between the curriculum-as-planned and the curriculum-as-lived experience. Kim knows she has an ethical responsibility to follow the curriculum that is suggested by the Ministry of Education, but she also knows her students and the context in which they live in the community, their homes, and the school. Similar to Aoki's (as cited in Pinar & Irwin, 2005) reference to another teacher, Miss O, "she knows that inevitably the quality of life lived within the tensionality depends much on the quality of the pedagogic being that she is" (Pinar & Irwin, 2005, p. 161). Kim was often frustrated about how the curriculum-as-planned was not attuned to the needs of this particular group of students and often at odds with her way of being a teacher. But Kim chose to just recognize this "tensionality in her pedagogical situation as a mode of being a teacher" (Aoki, as cited in Pinar & Irwin, 2005, p. 162), focused on who was in front of her, and tried to find balance in order to actively live the curriculum *with* the students, not merely deliver and install it. This allowed her to tap into her students' energies to consider new ideas and pedagogical ontologies to be creative, imaginative, and alive. Kumar's (2013) review of MacDonald's educational insights further clarifies that "it is the perceptive understanding of how one lives—thinks, feels, and acts—that constitutes learning rather than mere passive information absorption" (p. 100).

The two curriculum worlds appear somewhat dualistic if you look at teaching as an objective place you go to. Dwelling in between recognizes teaching as a way of *being*—who you are, the way you live life *is* your way of being a teacher. Inasmuch as there is a nondualism to living in between the two curriculum worlds, there is also no separation between personal and professional identities. I am always intrigued by the discussion regarding "work-life balance" as if they are two different entities separate from ourselves. Balance relates to wholeness and being able to pay attention to all aspects of *life*. Kim recognized that for her to be able to guide her students to live well requires her own balance—emotionally, spiritually, physically, and mentally. The added element of participating in this inquiry was a factor in her own wellness, thus we had to adjust accordingly. It meant I needed to ensure I asked and probed about her physical, spiritual, mental, and emotional wellbeing on a regular basis. Sometimes this meant cancelling observations or rescheduling our one-on-one discussions and other times it meant our conversations included time for "venting." I understood that she may need to clear what was swirling in her head—to acknowledge it and let it go, to be still and breathe before we could begin our dialogue about our inquiry. Over time we realized talking about her struggle to maintain balance also taught us something about what it means to live a curriculum of wellness.

A Mindful Journey Begins: *Currere*

As previously outlined in Chapter 3, the *currere* process was a series of guided writing exercises that assisted us in connecting educational issues with reflection of past, present (and future) personal and professional life events, artifacts, and other phenomena. Pinar (2004) outlines four steps in the method of *currere*: the regressive, progressive, analytical, and synthetical. The regressive moment constitutes past lived experience, both personal and social, where the teacher re-enters the past in order to transform memory to the present. In the progressive step, one looks toward the future to what is not yet, to future possibilities. In the analytic step, the past and present are examined to create subjective space, ultimately asking the question: "How is the future present in the past, the past in the future and the present in both?" (Pinar, 2004, p. 37). The synthetical involves re-entering the "lived present" and mindfully (re) conceptualizing the present experience.

We understood very quickly that this inquiry journey was clearly not a linear methodology where we finished one stage to be able to go onto the next. We decided to continue the *currere* process throughout the semester and because the synthetical involves re-entering the "lived present" and mindfully (re)conceptualizing the present experience, we believed that at the end of the semester, we could finish with the final *currere* writing focused on synthesis. In essence, as we reflected and revisited the regressive and progressive events and experiences initially identified in the summer months, we revealed multiple layers of meaning and significance as we lived the curriculum throughout the semester. Over time we could see and feel what became clear to be the key principles and philosophical grounding for Kim as a teacher and for the course. As an observer, I watched her relive her regressive and progressive moments with her students, and as a participant I experienced how it felt to learn from someone who was being and becoming incredibly self-aware, mindful, and connected. We met approximately every two weeks to discuss the key events, experiences, people, and places that were significant to the class. Discussions touched on a wide variety of topics such as curricular content, students, assessment practices, colleagues, afterschool events, school and/or district policy, parents, health, scheduling, stress, and political pressures. How she chose to navigate through these experiences constituted how she situated herself in the classroom and was a key piece to her way of being a teacher. We realized that this inquiry process was not just a combination of other methods; it went beyond. *Currere* and action research contributed greatly as a foundation; however, this was a unique mode of inquiry, wisdom-guided inquiry.

As an outsider working with teachers in their own classrooms, it is important to understand how difficult it is for teachers to engage in the inquiry process without feeling that research is being conducted *on* them, not *with* them. This sets up a power dynamic that is counterproductive to collaborative research, whereas within a "collaborative research stance, decision making is more of a shared process and insiders are part of the process in terms of assessing their own vulnerability as well as how to best return the data to the setting." (Herr & Anderson, 2005, p. 123). Teachers have an impressive amount of wisdom to offer, but so often there is an underlying apathy remaining from previous "outsider" projects (from policymakers, district researcher projects, etc.) during which the teachers' real thoughts and opinions are not necessarily heard. Sometimes processes are set up to record ideas on the surface but there is not ample time to build the necessary relationships to reveal the real questions behind the issues that are on the surface. This inquiry process could be another way to work with teachers to have the *complicated conversations* about teaching physical education. The *currere* process helps to build a strong collaborative relationship where there is continual negotiation to democratize the power relationships that exist with researcher and participant, knowledge and existing institutional tensions. In addition, as co-researchers, we needed to become comfortable with tensions. Practicing, living in the tensions *is* the true nature of this type of inquiry. An inquiry process with action research needs to be collaborative, democratic, and empowering. Winter (2003) explains, "only within a set of relationships which are experienced as 'empowering,' where there is a genuine sense of trust, mutual respect, equality and autonomy, will the inquiry be able to draw on all individuals' inherent creative potential" (p. 143). Facilitating and maintaining these relationships is the real work. From this, authentic and rich conversations emerge.

The remainder of this chapter will present highlights of our *currere* discussions, my own descriptions of pedagogical encounters as researcher-as-observer and researcher-as-participant, and some synthesis moments about the inquiry process. Together, these observations and analysis begin to provide a deeper understanding about the inquiry process and the complexities of living a curriculum of wellness.

The Regressive

The regressive stage focused on looking back at past experiences, people, and events that may have shaped our way(s) of thinking about teaching physical education. Pinar and Grumet (1976) explain:

> The biographical past exists presently.... While we say it cannot be held accountable for the present, the extent to which it is ignored is probably the extent it does account for what is present. Unconsciousness perpetuates itself. (p. 56)

Active and connected. A key foundation for Kim was her childhood way of life—being outdoors, active, playing in backyards, lakes, and at school. She felt connected to her body, to the land, to her family, and to the community of people around her. She has fond memories of the active and healthy way of life.

> *Growing up was always about playing outside at the family cabin, skipping, biking around the neighborhood, running track in the backyard, baseball in the backyard; we had a volleyball net; we played handball on our driveway, basketball, waterskiing, all that kind of stuff. So that's my memory of early childhood. Within school I remember starting school just loving it.... I had amazing elementary school teachers, very welcoming classrooms, and I remember loving recess.*

Compassion and kindness. Kim spoke about wanting to feel accepted and welcomed when she reflected on her autobiographical writings from stage one.

> *Whenever I'm in a room or anywhere, I, as a teacher, as a coach, as a friend, want everyone—every student, team member, family member—to feel that they're included, to feel wanted.*

This desire for acceptance originated from her experiences in junior high school where she was excluded by peer groups, alienated in physical education class, and stereotyped in sports. Kim believes that the result of these experiences is that she is kind and compassionate with students and people in general. Her level of empathy and ability to focus on building relationships are key pieces to how she is as a teacher.

> *I remember the creation of the cool group at school. I had been friends with all these girls and I had been popular and then the girls made a "cool group." It was the five prettiest girls and I wasn't in that. The rest of us were excluded and the boys voted on who was the hottest. They made a list and ranked us all out of 10…. To this day it really affected me…it affected my self-esteem, my body image.*

> *When I made the senior girls volleyball team it was the first time in 10 years that a grade 7 had made the senior team. My athlete friends deserted me because I was better than them and I remember going home crying. So I had to play down my talent a lot in Phys. Ed class. I deliberately missed shots and I wouldn't play my hardest because I didn't want to beat the boys because then I am even less of a female. And if I was too good on the sports field, the girls didn't like me. So I remember toning it down and trying not to be good. When basketball came around, they [coaches] said, "Keep it up—we need you." So I'm trying not to be good and then I'm trying to be the star all at the same time while trying to be pretty and impress the boys and impress everybody else.*

> *If I see someone being excluded at school, it kills me, it breaks my heart. So I always try in all my classes to get everyone involved, especially in my Phys. Ed classes. I always mix it up and get them to talk about their weekends, find someone who went to the same junior high…because to be to left out in a class every day for five months and not talk to anyone is so awful.*

While kindness and compassion are positive characteristics for teachers to possess, they have to be careful in their approach to providing only to the collective other. Kim recognized that it was and is incredibly difficult to maintain balance and ensure you are taking care of yourself. Without a focus on your own health, without connecting body, mind, and spirit, you actually become less able to contribute positively to your community. Living with compassion and kindness does not mean giving your energy away to others; rather, it is about merging your energy with others and the universe.

Kim understands now that her desire to be accepted and always wanting to accommodate everyone, while beneficial for being empathetic to her students, also drove her to a most unhealthy state. Kim's struggle was taking care of herself while trying to live a kind and compassionate life. Achieving that balance requires us to be connected, to be still, to be mindful. So many of Kim's past events and experiences did not honor her own self, what was best for her; rather, it was often about what was best for her coaches, teachers, students, parents, friends, teammates, and classmates. This led to what we often see with many physical education teachers—a frantic, chaotic schedule of coaching, organizing tournaments, intramurals, activity events, coordinating off-site physical education activities, and full-time teaching. She wanted to provide leadership and make a difference in her athletes' and students' lives, but the more she did, the faster the pace, the greater the responsibility and pressure, and the more unhealthy she became.

> It was extremely stressful being a traveling teacher—you're in Phys. Ed then you're rushing to a social studies class, you're booking venues, you are trying to book buses, you are all over the place. Then practice would start at 3:30. I would be in class and I would be planning my practice because I was barely staying afloat, just barely keeping up…not eating, not sleeping, I started grinding my teeth horribly and feeling very isolated. The coaching took over—I felt like a coach teaching on the side.

> Then I had a car accident that changed everything forever and I hit rock bottom. I should have stopped coaching because the pain, headaches, and stress but I kept going.… I was not in a good place at all. I was so miserable, I just wanted to sleep, get a sub, but I couldn't because I had a team. I had to be at practice every day so I couldn't miss school and show up for practices.

Eventually Kim stopped coaching competitive extracurricular sport and focused on her own ill health. She believes at that point only a catastrophic event such as a car accident could make her pay attention to what she was doing to her overall long-term health.

> I think it was the universe's way of saying, "you are stubborn and you're never going to quit all of this, so boom!" I was at rock bottom. I just know that if I was still doing all of that [coaching] today I would not be healthy and happy. I would still be doing it, it would be my whole life, but I think the universe knew that I was stubborn and it was going to take quite the hard landing to make me snap out of it.

At this point Kim began to use more holistic ways to live her life, manage her pain, and reconnect to her body. She enrolled in evening yoga sessions and belly dance and eventually got certified in Hatha yoga. She began to practice meditation and guided relaxation, and shifted her teaching focus to holistic ways of being active. It is important to note that letting go of her coaching lifestyle was very difficult.

> Admitting you are weak and admitting you can't do something is devastating but the biggest lesson I tell people is just because you're good at something doesn't mean you should do it.

And I was a very good coach, no, an excellent coach. I don't want to sound like I'm tooting my own horn but I was an amazing coach. What I did with this program, what I did, very few people have done. But it was killing me. I just knew that the stress was going to eventually kill me. I remember a quote, "stress can be the equivalent of eating 2 Big Macs a day" —the wear and tear on your arteries and your system…it's abusing your body physically. I knew I had to step back from coaching, and now that I have, now I see people and they say, you look younger, you look so relaxed or "boy, you look good." I never knew how during the 10 years I coached I looked so horrible.

I still run the tournament and I get to see all my old coaching friends—that's what I probably missed the most, that camaraderie. I now sponsor the volleyball team, so I'm still involved but it is hard—knowing that I was one of the best and stepping away. I remember coaches saying, "you just finished second in the province, why are you quitting coaching?" How do you explain that? It wasn't easy but they see me now and they say I look great. And I say, yes, because I'm not that coach pulling her hair out on the side of the court, screaming, veins popping out of my head. I just shifted that energy. I'm still coaching but I am coaching yoga. And I'm coaching life skills and coaching those types of things that I think are way more valuable for students…and I think I'm reaching a grander audience. Instead of reaching 12 athletes a year, I'm now reaching 60–90 Holistic Health Option students a year and passing on those great messages.

Taking this further, there is a fine line when taking care of others as to when it can become detrimental to your own self. Kim's struggle was balancing her life so she was able to take care of herself while being kind and compassionate. We discussed this idea of taking care of others further and how this can either be positive energy or turn into a health crisis.

When I think of my coaching days…it's so addictive, it's like heroine—wanting to win, wanting to be the best. Before life was much simpler, playing, being outside with [brother] and growing up at the cabin. It's hard to believe that was the same girl.

Balance. When she was a young child, Kim found the balance in playing with her non-athlete friend, being active with her brother, being unplugged.

I was a very good athlete at a very young age. But my next-door neighbor was in a different school district and the total "non-athlete." She was the exact opposite of me. So I would come home from this intense practice with all this pressure and then we would just go play Barbies or dress-up. It was such a good balance for me and she just always kept me grounded. I love that because I think I would have become a "basketball head," it would've totally narrowed me. She helped me with that. She didn't care if we lost a national championship and she would say, "oh, you did so well!" At the end of the day that's what really matters, I think. Even when you watch the Olympics—they train for four years, and look,

Simon Whitfield just fell off his bike, and if you have nothing else to fall back on, if he doesn't have family friends, so that's why I'm glad I had a balance.

Coaching as an asset. As a high-level coach, Kim admits to her initial focus being highly competitive in a performance-based world. The challenge is paying attention to how coaching influences your teaching and who you are as a teacher. Coaching needs to be an asset to teaching, enhancing and positively influencing your program, rather than a detriment. Coaches push athletes to be their best but you have to understand this looks different in the classroom, in physical education.

Being competitive—I had to bring it down a few notches because you just lose them otherwise…. So in my social studies classes along with my Phys. Ed class, I tell my students—I don't remember all the games, I don't remember what my stats were, but I remember the people and I remember the experiences so school should be about the people.

Kim felt the leadership, compassion, organization, and dedication you have to have as a coach are important traits to bring to teaching and you have to figure out how this can make you a better teacher, a better person. Often the competitive, skill-based focus of the coaching world finds its way into the high school physical education setting, but Kim's experience as an athlete and a varsity coach led her to having a different outlook on teaching.

I rode the bench for three years and all of a sudden I was voted captain. I would put notes in everybody's locker—everybody (not just the starters). I remember one girl logged one minute and 17 seconds that whole year and we ended up winning the national championship that year. And when the buzzer went, that girl was jumping on the bench screaming, it would have been so easy for her to not feel part of the team that year and to have quit, and you know you get the bench players who hate the starters but we just have that group. I just made everybody feel important because I have been a bench player.

I didn't start in the national final—I probably played two minutes in the game but I knew that I had a huge part of that victory. So as a physical educator that was always my approach…it doesn't matter how much talent you have, it's those intangibles. So coming out of Pandas basketball, my greatest asset to the team wasn't my scoring or my rebounding or my defense; it was my ability to lead and include people and make everybody feel like they mattered. It's all tone, it's all how you set the stage.

A work in progress—practicing. Kim spoke about how with her disciplined and "be the best" background, she has to consciously remind herself to slow down, relax, and manage her stress.

It's always a work in progress for me to slow down.… I used to be so high strung. It was a huge lesson for me to just relax a little bit. Whenever I start going back, I take a breath. I actually started a rule when I was a traveling teacher. I wouldn't start my class until 5 minutes after the bell. You [students] can open up a book and you can talk but I need 5 minutes because I would get to class and I would be rushed and stressed. And if you come into a class like that, that is the mood you are setting for the whole 80 minutes. I have to work at meditation, I have to work at calming myself down to sleep, I have to work at when I'm caught in traffic, to breathe. And when a student swears at you…I just remember to breathe and not take it personally.

Lifestyle—a way of life.

It has been a good lesson for my students—how I climbed out of my unhealthy situation with holistic remedies, changing my schedule, getting rid of my stressors, breathing, and getting into noncompetitive activities. Belly dancing, yoga—there's no winner and I love that. My friend asked me why I don't play competitive women's basketball and I say, "Never! It's just not good for me." And will I coach again? I don't know. It's so far off for me right now. I'm so happy. Lionel [husband], he was never a high-level athlete, he played basketball and he bowled but it wasn't something super intense. I get home and he says "let's go for a bike ride, let's go for a walk." Those are the activities where you stay active and finding someone who keeps you active. I'm healthier than I ever have been before, and happier, and I think it shows in my teaching—in my social studies class and my Phys. Ed class.

It's about living life—it's not about the compartments of coaching or teaching, this or that. It's helping your students understand that it's not just about what's in the classroom; it's about how you live your life. It doesn't stop when the bell rings. You have to be a good person and it's not easy.

Relationships. Kim spoke about her time as a teacher when she was at the peak of her coaching stress and how this did not allow for enough time for her to know her students and for her students to get to know her. It was easy to build relationships with her athlete-students because she was with them for so many hours in the week, but the majority of students in such classes often feel marginalized, alienated.

I did not have relationships with my students because it was survival. I was barely, barely breathing. You just go, survivor mode. So now I think I take the time to let my students know me.… When I first started teaching, I never let them into my personal life. Even me putting pictures up of myself—this is a whole new thing for me. I never displayed my personal life at school. I kept it very separate. So my students didn't know me, they probably thought I slept under my desk! I think me just opening up more and putting up pictures and letting them know who I am. It's not that I tell everything to my students, I just say this and that, and then they open up a little bit more.

The Progressive

In the progressive stage, there are no limits to the vision that a teacher may have, we look "at what is not yet the case, what is not yet present" (Pinar & Grumet, 1976, p. 58). Kim looked at her teaching, her relationships with students and colleagues, her emotional and intellectual projections, and imagined and described a future several years from now. The following summarizes the imagined future state of her class, students, school, and education system.

Stillness and meditation. Kim's vision for the future begins with the idea of stillness and starting/finishing the day with a time where everyone in the school is "unplugged" and can slow down for a moment.

> I would like to see on a school-wide basis starting with a daily meditation for all students. For 5 or 10 minutes, you get to school and everybody gets focused at the beginning of the day. Starting out with volunteers a few mornings and it grows and grows to where it gets to all staff and students. Do a little timeout and focus at the beginning of the day...mindfulness.

Teachers and students within class time, especially physical education, can benefit greatly with this focus because it gives time not only for stillness and letting go of the day or week's events, but an opportunity to connect body-mind-spirit as an individual and to each other to build relationships.

> I think starting out Phys. Ed classes and ending it with meditation would be good. Start the class with the meditation and finish it with some stretching, a cool down and just a reflection on how your body feels. Just more awareness not just show up, participate, leave, but more of a "hey, how are you doing today? And are we eating well?" I do a food blog with my Phys. Ed classes. I call it a healthy habit log book. I don't think a lot of Phys. Ed teachers focus a lot on students' eating habits, how they are sleeping, what they are drinking or any other patterns like that. In the healthy habit logbook, they log their habits for a week and there is even a box in the corner where they draw a picture of their emotions' so how they're feeling—a happy face or a sad face. They log what they are eating, how they exercise, and how they are sleeping every day. All of them tell me how helpful that is.

Beyond the school. Kim broadened her vision beyond her own school to a systemic viewpoint and described a minimum two-option physical education program model.

> In 5 or 10 years, I see "Phys. Ed 10–Holistic Health" and a "Phys. Ed 10-Sport." I have run what I call a Phys. Ed 10–Holistic Health where I do the sports...today's basketball and then do yoga in the studio. And then we'll go back and do another day of basketball and then

do belly dancing. So even the students who don't like basketball are still going to show up for that "unit" because two of the five days we are in the studio doing something else.

While visionary and optimistic in this progressive reflection exercise, it was difficult for her to continue this type of thinking without tempering it with the political realities of the education system.

It has to start with Alberta Ed., the universities and teacher education, so maybe we are talking 20 years by that time. And I think just individual schools...I created this holistic health option by myself, so others could too. That's why starting it at the university level and government can be slow and frustrating. So starting at the universities and just teaching it in this way... because we have flexibility in the curriculum.

Teacher autonomy. While Kim's vision for the future of physical education includes official programing changes, she also believes that with any curriculum, teachers have the freedom to make professional decisions on their own.

I think it isn't the content, it's the interpretation. It's the teachers that we have to work on because I am taking that curriculum and just bending it within limits. I think I'm having a lot of success and I'm sure [some] would argue that girls aren't going on to take Phys Ed. Well, a lot of them are going on to take holistic health.... You will get two or three girls in a Phys Ed 20 or 30 class and the rest of them are taking holistic health.... I think it's just another option and something that they are interested in and it's not that competitive. I am still doing Phys. Ed 10 but just in a different manner with a slightly different focus.

Making connections in higher education. Kim further elaborates on the university teacher education programs and the instructors' contribution to making this vision happen.

University instructors—what are they emphasizing? Are they aware of mindfulness and a holistic approach? Are the students eating, sleeping—are student teachers checking in with kids at the beginning of class? It should go without saying, but I know as a first-year teacher, you get to class, quickly take the attendance, and you go! So just teaching them [student teachers] to slow down. A lot of them have an 80-minute class—there is time to check in at the beginning, there's time to do a good warm-up, or a meditation at the beginning of class.... I don't want this to be a secret; I don't want this to be that I am the only one doing this. More people need to do it and more people just need to be aware.

Student wellness. The rationale for a wellness-oriented approach in high school physical-education programing is also a significant piece to Kim's future scenario. She recognizes the growing dilemma for our children in an information age where instant gratification and quick fixes contribute to an unhealthy, unsustainable pace for many young people.

> Life is getting faster and it [Holistic Health Option] is the perfect counterbalance to slow down. All four classes, the kids have their cell phones on them all day. In other Phys. Ed classes, they're tucked into their sports bras; they have them underneath their desk in social and math. But in Holistic Health they don't bring their phones to class and if they do they're at the back of the room in their bags on silent. That speaks volumes that they are putting down their phones during class. That is one of the biggest compliments—that during class a cell phone never goes off in my room. They honestly shut down. That 80 minutes is the longest they will go all day without their cell phones.

Beyond the self. Part of Kim's progressive writing included imagining how she would like to be remembered when she finishes her teaching career, thus allowing her to think about how she, as a teacher, has transformed herself and impacted others.

> I was officially recognized by the Alberta Health and Physical Education Council with the Certificate of Commendation. When I first got that award I was a little embarrassed.... I don't like the idea of "'you're better teacher than this person, you are better than her." People were coming up to me and congratulating me... my answer to them was I'm just happy that people are talking about the Holistic Health Option class.

> So in the future if I get recognized or if the course gets recognized or it becomes part of the curriculum in any way shape or form.... I just want more people doing it. But how do you put it into words and that is why you are here doing this. So having people contact me on how to do this scares me a little bit...so then we're back to how do we teach them to do what we're doing.

Focus on the students. A key part of Kim's impetus for this course is not the vision for the program, school, or future students, but her current students' future. She says to her students:

> There is going to come a time when you don't even remember any of your teachers' names, none of the kids who you went to school with. So although you think that this is the biggest thing in your life, you have 60 more years to live after you leave the school—maybe 70 or 80. So how are you going to do this? I love telling the kids how old I am, although it makes me cry sometimes. I hope they remember thinking back when I'm doing a circuit with them and it's not easy—we do a Tabata circuit and I almost die—hopefully they'll say, "Wow, she was 35 and she was kicking ass in that circuit or she was belly dancing or she was doing yoga." I like telling them where I am at, how I got here, and get them to think about the rest of their lives. For the grade 10s, after [taking] my class, they can't fit another Holistic Health

Option class into their timetable because they don't have room in their schedule but they're going to get a membership, join the Y, or do yoga with their mom, or they buy a yoga mat for home. Those are the things where I'm thinking okay, you've learned. Their reflections at the end of the course, they tell me that they've learned how to eat, I'm nicer to my parents, I don't gossip anymore. It's about those little lessons. I like modeling and them seeing into the future. We do vision boards with them—where they are going to be in 5 years, 10 years, 20 years, 30 years. It freaks them out but it gets them thinking about how they're going to stay healthy and active.

Analysis

The *currere* analysis phase involves describing the present with the biographical information that has come forward inclusive of responses to the past and future (Pinar & Grumet, 1976). This involves describing what ideas, events, people, places, experiences, and emotions we are drawn to. "Description via conceptualization is breaking into parts the organic whole" (Pinar & Grumet, 1976, p. 59). Kim and I began the analysis phase of *currere* in the summer before classes started.

Traditional action research models describe the process as being a series of spirals that are comprised of information gathering, analysis, reflection, and action. Interestingly, the *currere* process uses the same types of elements within an autobiographical stance. Each time we let in what freely comes to our consciousness and reflect and record it into autobiographical text, we in essence acquire biographical information that can move us in a nonlinear, multidimensional way. Pinar explains (1976):

If I write about my biographic situation as I see it (not as I *want* to see it, although this can be included) then it is as if I have escaped from it. It is *there*, on the paper in a way, and I am still here, at the typewriter, looking at the print and the conceptualization of the perspective that *was* mine, and so the place is new. (Pinar & Grumet, 1976, p. 52)

The following collection of the conversations between us captures Kim's analysis of the regressive and progressive as she saw it before the semester began. It would prove to be just the beginning, as the course continued to (un)fold with an unpredictable nonlinear temporality that provided further opportunities for growth and evolution. As Wang (2010) explains, "more layers are added to *currere's* temporal complexity as each synthesis opens up rather than converges toward an authentic self. *Currere* becomes an ongoing process of unlearning, learning and education" (p. 282).

Currere analysis: Kim's highlights

I want everyone to feel included as a teacher, as a coach, as a friend, I want to be remembered. I want to make an impact, so don't just be here but be here on the planet and do something. I was always an old soul so even when I was younger, I would think about what would my parents think, what will I think about this in 10 years or 20 years...very mature with that and I think nowadays kids are just in the now. That's why I'm teaching holistic habits. They don't care about 20 years from now what their arteries are going to look like. They don't care about their behaviour.

An over-riding theme is my concern for other people, pleasing others. And I'm still trying to overcome that.

There's so much stuff so it's hard to just choose one thing but wanting to feel accepted and welcomed was big.

What I am most proud of is the national championships with the Pandas, my first year as a coach, winning a national championship. Those things but also getting home and realizing there's only 15 people that really care about that championship. Outside that team there's probably 15 people that actually care you won a national championship. That was always very hard and that's why I had to get out of it, it was killing me. You don't do it for recognition but for the amount of hell I was going through and no one cared, I wondered how it really mattered in the world. But then I get married and everyone cares. So for me it's the people.

I'm also most proud of being a great friend. My ability to bring people together on and off the court, and as a coach I could unite people and make everyone feel like they're a part of the victory/loss. And at my wedding, all different people coming together. That's what I'm proud of.

When I think of what I would have done differently...hitting rock bottom. It still makes me sick thinking about it. But of course, 20/20 hindsight now that my life is happier and I can look back at that person and say, "why did you do that?" I'm absolutely mortified that it got to that point of me not taking a sick day in that whole year. And for what, because I had to coach a high school basketball team! That was more important than my health. What? I still feel horrible—obviously I can hardly talk about it and look you in the eye when I'm talking about it. But now, that is what happened, I see it was me putting everybody else ahead.

M: Did that incident, that period of time do anything for you moving forward?

K: So I won a city championship (which is twisted). But we win city championship, finished second at provincials—the best finish this school has ever had and I took five weeks off and I got better. I rested that entire summer and I came back with a better holistic health program and a studio.

M: But as a teacher, as a person, not your accomplishments, not the tangible things...

K: *Forgiving yourself. Because forgiveness is something I try to tell my students. We do a spirituality stream, laughter yoga, compassion, mindfulness, and Fridays is for forgiveness. I had always thought that forgiveness was for other people and we never forgive ourselves. So I had to forgive myself. You forgive your friends easily but we don't forgive ourselves.*

M: *So what did that allow you to do then?*

K: *To go on, to move forward. Actually, I just figured out forgiveness...because for years I was teaching holistic health saying forgive other people and a guest instructor said the hardest person to forgive is yourself. That was just in June and I realized I had forgiven everyone else but I hadn't really truly forgiven myself.*

M: *The way that you have now framed it I see that as one of the positive things in your life.*

K: *I'm not quite there yet*

M: *I think if you hadn't really hit that rock bottom, you really wouldn't have stopped and taken stock—you'd still be coaching, you'd still be beating up your own body, you'd still be disconnected and going 100 miles an hour and you wouldn't be healthy*

K: *Yes, but do we really need these hard lessons? But I think I have a harder head—the universe has to hit me harder to get my attention.*

Another theme...being excluded, being left out, being told you're not good enough, cool enough, pretty enough. That empathy I have for other kids going through that.

So when I think about whether I see anything I was angry about.... I'm not an angry person—I use my anger to motivate me in a positive way. I don't have the patience to wait around for other people to get this [a new program of study] passed and go through all the paperwork so I'll just do it myself. And now I have three sections again, it's flying.

I look back at my thoughts on coaching and have mixed emotions—I have my little wall there, all my former players, it's just great memories. When they heard that I got married they were cheering—you know that love from great athletes who understood me.

So I know for me walking through the school, every cell phone I would stop and every hat violation. I was wearing myself out being the moral police for everybody. I think I have a very strong sense of who I am. My mom wouldn't let it go.... So that's how I grew up and my dad, same thing, so both of my parents are very opinionated, they will never change their mind on something.... That's how we grew up.... But so now I do forgive and forget.

And when I make my mind up and when it comes to excluding people, picking on people, mistreating people, I have zero tolerance and my students know that. You do not make a racial slur in my class—it's not funny, it's not allowed. So my past, I always refer back to my past, strong teachers, strong parents. But sometimes…it would be nice to just hang out in the background.

Day to day, I want to be happy—that's my mantra, every day for the rest of my life, and that guides me in the decisions I'm making today—to stop coaching, to not return to coaching, to distance myself from negative people, start the fun patrol at school, to meditate, to do yoga, my decision to marry Lionel. I know every day we are so happy—he is sweet medicine to me. And I don't want to end up crippled with arthritis so I'm physically looking after myself. I'm not carrying baggage—our stress is carried here and that's where a lot of people carry their stress. I just want to be healthy and happy. I want to let go of grudges and forgive and I do forgive a lot more than I used to. Everything, if I do something…is that really going to make me happy? If not and it's negative energy, is that going to help? So the past molds me but now I do think a lot about the future and just whom I want to be with and where I want to go and whom I want to be with.

M: You said it before, the courage it takes to step up…it's harder to stay healthy, it sounds funny but it's easier to stay unhealthy…

K: Way easier, but teachers…we just keep going and we get sick. But now for me I will take days off. I could push myself to get through but I now say no, I'm looking after myself. Those who never take a sick day for 40 years, at the end of it are you really that healthy?

A Mindful Journey Continues

When classes began so too did our journey as co-researchers *living* the inquiry process. Every week, I attended at least two H2O classes where I participated, observed, and reflected on my experiences and/or observations. I wrote about class routines; technical information; daily activities; Kim's actions, words, questions, and ideas; possible connections to Kim's past, present, and future thoughts; and sometimes my own experiences as a participant. These notes and reflections became part of our ongoing discussions and ultimately contributed to our understanding of how to teach in this way. It is important to note that my observations and reflections were brought forward in a way that would maintain the collaborative relationship. We had built a level of trust throughout the first stages of *currere* that was to be respected, and I realized that some issues needed to be handled delicately. In essence, this meant that it might be weeks before we addressed what I observed and/or experienced. The following section provides my interpretation and perceptions about the H2O course from the point of view of participant and observer. Unfortunately, I am unable to capture via text the energy and essence that was present in the class but vitally important to understanding what it means to teach in a holistic and wellness-oriented way. Perhaps an exercise in futility, the intent is to describe the atmosphere, activities, interactions, and movements within the class, as well as Kim's way of teaching, so that individuals are better able to understand the process we lived to co-construct meaning.

The home base for H2O was a classroom that had been converted to a studio. On one side of the room there were large windows that provided significant natural light that allowed Kim to turn off the florescent lights, which she did on a regular basis. Outside the windows were trees and grass, and Kim added numerous indoor plants at the back of the room. On another wall were floor-to-ceiling mirrors—very helpful for physical activity instruction where students can self-check their form and technique, and the teacher can monitor and give feedback. The teaching space also included a white board, teacher desk, file cabinet, and some shelving. Kim made a specific effort to de-clutter the room and created a welcome environment with inspirational banners, posters, and pictures. These were the physical characteristics of the room. What could not be seen, however, is the energy in this room—positive energy, love, support, and a sense of calm. Her wall was filled with photos of students, physical activity sessions, family, trees, scenery from her family's cabin—these together provided a snapshot of who Kim is. This seemingly small level of vulnerability would prove to be a key ingredient to teaching in a wellness-oriented way.

On the white board, Kim outlined each day with a theme:

Monday—"Marvel"

Tuesday—"Take a new perspective"

Wednesday—"Welcome kindness"

Thursday—"Thank you"

Friday—"Forgiveness"

Weekends—"Are for chocolate!"

On the first day, Kim briefly outlined the course and how it fit within the physical education department, and then immediately dove into the flow of the class. She talked about mindfulness, kindness—how we treat ourselves and others, and about paying attention, being aware. She emphasized non-competitiveness, nonperfection, discouraged students from comparing themselves to others, and encouraged patience (with self and others). She also asked students about how many of them ate breakfast and those who did not, she did not scold; she asked the class to share some common reasons that people do not eat breakfast. This opened up a discussion among teenagers about what was *behind* the issue. These students know that breakfast is important and Kim knew she did not have to tell them this. She was sympathetic—commenting that she has sometimes missed breakfast, and she was caring—communicating the message that she was concerned about each and every student's health. They then brainstormed organizing tips for easy breakfasts and how to support each other to make sure all came to school well-nourished and rested.

I was immediately struck by how engaged students were from the beginning of class to the end. All were listening; there was laughter at times and a sense of calm. It was clear that Kim was comfortable sharing her own stories about some of her experiences and willing to listen to her students to get a sense of what their worlds are like. She asked the students to describe their day-to-day activities, which painted a picture of the modern teenager's life: cell phones, social media, afterschool jobs, sports teams, clubs, television watching, self-judgment, meeting parental expectations, exams, marks, rankings, saving money for college/university, and somewhere in all of this, being healthy and active. This is where she introduced them to yoga—the teenager's "time-out" but at the same time learning movement flows and techniques that are grounded in philosophy that is focused on connecting body, mind, and spirit. This is one of the only opportunities during the school day where students get to "unplug," to stop for a moment, to pay attention, to be still. While it was a short introduction of a simple flow series, we were all focused on the body movements and our breath. We ended with what is called Savasana, "corpse pose," where you must lie still for several minutes. Kim warned us that this would take practice because it is very difficult for people to lie completely still and quiet our minds in our very busy worlds. "So, be patient and kind to yourselves," she said, "this is about practicing, and each day we get to start fresh and try again."

As a participant-observer, I flipped between experiencing the class and stepping outside for moments to observe and notice not only what I was doing but also what was going on around me. At the beginning of class, I watched and observed, taking note of the way Kim is, what she is doing and how she is with her students. I observed the students, their actions, how they respond to Kim, their overall attitude when they walk in the room. One of the first things I noticed was that there was never an issue with students not wearing appropriate clothing and rarely were students late. Kim greeted students as they came in and depending on the scheduled activity, students gathered materials and set up the equipment on their own, without prompting. Students helped each other know what to do. While there are often administrative tasks to do at the beginning of class, most of the time, Kim was able to accomplish these and still connect with several students on a personal level—asking them about their day, what they did on the weekend, and how their breakfast eating was going. Often Kim would start the class with a story about an experience from the day or week that challenged her in maintaining her healthy habits. I think students were surprised to hear that their physical education teacher is human and sometimes eats poorly and skips workouts. It was important for them to hear these types of stories because there is so much messaging for adolescents about being perfect. Other times, Kim would ask students to share their stories and if the energy in the room was low, she'd say "who's got a positive story today? We need some positive energy in the room." As a participant, it was amazing to feel the transformation that happens when excitement and positive energy is shared among youth—it creates an atmosphere that is welcoming, a place you want to be.

Every week, Kim posted the schedule of activities for the following week, so that students begin to have some stability and know what to expect. This semester, Kim purposefully scheduled yoga for Mondays. Instilling this idea of regular mindful practice connects to the philosophical grounding of yoga. Every Monday students know that they will be practicing yoga, allowing them to focus their thoughts, acknowledge their weekend activities and let go, and set an intention for the day or the week.

In the first few weeks as participant-observer, I realized that this consistent yoga practice was a key piece to a wellness-oriented approach. It became apparent that it was not the actual yoga activity itself—different poses, flows, posture, flexibility—it was the principles of mindfulness, connection, and nonpermanence that are key us, individually and collectively, being healthy and well. One morning she began the class,

Your body is thanking you for taking this time…a reminder to take a few moments every day for you…to find the positive energy within and around you, to let go of the stressors in your life and focus on just breathing for a moment.

She taught the class how to set our minds to the present, return to the breath if our mind wanders and focus on postures in the moment—connecting body, mind, and spirit. She guided us in mindful practice, drawing our attention to the energy in our body, breathing in positive energy and exhaling anything that does not serve us; encouraging us to follow every breath and pay attention to what is happening in all parts of our body. Perhaps our arms feel light, maybe our toes are throbbing, our fingers tingling, shoulders tight, jaw clenched—be aware of what's going on. She told a personal story about how balancing poses are like a barometer for her. If she skips breakfast, is not getting enough sleep, has too many things on her plate, she rarely can hold a balance pose. In other words, she knows that her life is not in balance and this draws her attention to it so that she can make the adjustments. She also uses it in preparation for dance performances, games, etc. She knows that if she cannot hold a balance pose beforehand, she is not connected and needs to focus her thoughts, let go, and breathe.

Consistently, Kim used humor and personal stories to maintain the welcoming and inclusive atmosphere in the class. For example, the day she introduced belly dancing she explained,

My first belly dancing class in the community, I was the worst belly dancer my instructor had ever seen! But I knew I needed to do something because my hips were locked up. My mom just had a hip replacement and I didn't want to see that happen for me. The music, the costumes, finger cymbals, it was so fun. And yes, it helped my hips but it has taught me how to love my body. I have never been able to touch my toes, I sucked at gymnastics, I'm boxy and tall but it doesn't matter, any shape or size can belly dance. It's all about jiggling and the more I jiggle, the better. I just love it! I put my hip scarf on and vacuum the house in it—it's awesome! [Giggles throughout the room]

Kim's attitude and relationality with students characterizes and sets the tone of the class. On this particular occasion, Kim concluded the introduction to belly-dancing class with a reminder about accepting the body we have and ended with a hug to the self.

A key activity that students do is called the "Healthy Habits Log Book" (HHLB). They start by reflecting and describing their own health, as well as monitoring their daily habits for a week. While a snapshot, Kim explains that there is a real discrepancy between students' perception of their health habits and their actual habits. They record sleep patterns, nutrition, water intake, exercise, stress, and overall emotional health. Kim has students discuss their ideas about all these components to determine their level of knowledge. Again, high school students know a significant amount of correct information but mention their frustration with the onslaught of information in the media that makes it confusing. Kim reviews evidence-based nutritional knowledge with a key message about moderation, research about sleep patterns, and dieting, and reminds students on how to choose appropriate information sources on the internet.

When students completed their HHLBs and returned them to Kim, she reviewed all of them and provided opportunity for discussion. Students discussed what they noticed, what surprised them, what they would like to improve upon, where they could get more information. They also gave each other feedback and asked Kim for advice. What I noticed is how the tone of the discussion was not judgmental. The purpose was not to lecture students about what they *should* be doing; it was an open discussion about the challenges of real life for these students and sharing solutions and information about alternatives. For example, if students talked about how difficult they find it is to eat a healthy lunch, instead of discussing "what is a healthy lunch?" the issues behind the question had to do with setting priorities, time management, peer influences, convenience, affordability, and skipping meals. They then began to share ideas about how to change habits when faced with such challenges.

Another course activity relates to Kim's belief about role modeling. It is important to her that she is a good role model for students not only for the present but to connect how she lives her life as a 35-year-old and where her students might be 20 years from now. So she walks them through a vision board activity where they gaze into their futures. She explains,

> Where are they going to be in 5, 10, 20, 30, 40 years? It freaks them out but it gets them thinking about how they want to, how they're going to stay healthy and active.

This assignment was well received by students and was important throughout the semester, as Kim was able to refer to their visions for their future when talking about the present, which made activities more relevant and meaningful.

Students also participated in different types of circuit training, including Tabata, cardiovascular, endurance, and strength-based circuits. In the first month, Kim gradually introduced students to Tabata, a high-intensity interval-training workout that can be completed in 20 minutes. She emphasized to the class, "I love this work-out! You can do this at home, on vacation, anywhere. It will be hard but short—this will be about your attitude and outlook. But remember, we're all here and in this together." During the session, she again used personal stories and drew attention to my struggle to complete the intervals, which provided another example of role modeling and a way to demonstrate to students that we are not perfect, but at 35 and 43 years of age we are still trying to maintain a healthy lifestyle. At the end of these particular classes, Kim encouraged students and told them how well they did. She asked them how they *felt* and they commented about how they did not think they could do it but because the intervals were only 20 seconds "you can get through it." There was also discussion about mood, energy, endorphins, and class support. Equally important to this lesson activity is how Kim connected it to the community and potential life-worlds of her students. She explained how this session was what you would typically see in a community recreation center or private fitness club. This is critical for adolescents who are very conscious about their bodies and sometimes have unrealistic perceptions about community fitness and recreation facilities. This discussion helps build their confidence to perhaps attend classes outside of the school environment.

Another day, a guest instructor was invited to lead students through a Zumba® class. Zumba® is a workout that combines Latin music and dance fitness movements. I participated in this class with students and found the introductory class quite advanced and the instructor quite difficult to follow. Afterwards I felt somewhat defeated, as I was not picking up on all the moves quickly enough. Many of us spent our time just doing "step-touch" and marching so as not to bump into other students. It was clear that many of us did not achieve the level of workout that the instructor did and I wondered how this element of the popular culture of the fitness industry promoted holistic health. I know we all heard the music but there was so much emphasis on coordinating the moves, it was difficult to enjoy "moving to the music." While not a new issue in physical and health education, often the challenge with community instructors is their knowledge (or lack of knowledge) of appropriate progressions for teaching children and youth in a school setting, which is not the same as instructing adults in recreation and fitness facilities.

At the end of the first month of classes, students participated in fitness testing. Students are measured in all health-related components of fitness using the following tests: Leger shuttle run, push-ups, sit-ups, back extension, flexibility, and lateral side-to-side line touch. Kim was very diligent about preparing students mentally for this fitness test day. She emphasized noncompetition:

This is all about you. This is individual, not about how you compare to others. This is just as much a mental test as it is physical so those who are waiting, be supportive of each other by cheering. Remember, nice big yoga breathing.

Afterwards, she again encouraged students and told them how proud she was of them. As I observed this testing day, I began to question its purpose and whether it was consistent with the philosophy of the course. I wondered about using objective performance measures and how it fits in with overall wellness. Should this type of fitness test be used to measure students' health and wellness? How does this connect to a holistic, wellness-oriented approach to teaching?

The schedule of topics and activities for October included yoga, line dancing, body flow workouts, Zumba®, hip-hop dancing, belly dancing, Reiki, guest speaker (Georgette Reed), Tabata, fitness circuits, a fitness center workout, Moksha yoga, Pilates, activities with grade 1 buddies, and interactive activities with Community Learning Skills Program students.

The first class of October began with Kim reminding us about using and bringing our own water bottles. During this discussion, focus was not only on the health benefits of drinking water regularly but also about how our own actions (not purchasing plastic water bottles) are connected to the overall health of the planet. The majority of the students who brought water that day (half the class) had their own water bottles. Interestingly, I noticed my own habits changing as a result of this regular practice. When preparing for my visits to class, my own personal water bottle was on my list to take—I knew it was not an option to stop and buy water. It extended beyond my class visits and became a part of my everyday routine. Every time I thought about buying a bottle of water, I remembered what we were trying to do in class and my consumption of bottled water declined to almost nothing. I found myself looking for water fountains, getting water from the tap, and not leaving the house without a full bottle of water. I was amazed at how the social culture of this one class had made such a difference.

Because this was a Monday, Kim also introduced the week's events and what to expect. We would be line dancing, belly dancing, learning about how to do a body-weight flow workout, and this particular day was yoga. Up until this class, yoga was taught by Kim and students generally followed. Today she began to talk about some principles of yoga, "I want you to start wrapping your head around yoga so you can do it at home, every day if you want to." She discussed how to put together a flow sequence themselves using some simple organizing points: front, side, back bends and twists; as well as sitting, kneeling, standing, stomach, and back. Very gently, she also explained what it meant when we have our hands open—we are exchanging energy from ourselves to/ from the universe, and when we put our palms/fingers together as we do in the Namaste position it induces calmness.

As I participated in the yoga class that day, I noted how thankful I was to be there as my weekend's events had been challenging. I always found the energy in the room supportive. It was not all about it being positive; it was understanding that there is a commonality among all of us—our struggles, pain, triumphs, and joy—it is all there but with no labels or judgments, it is just in the room and something about that connection to each other is incredibly powerful yet calming. I reflected,

> I truly believe that what I'm experiencing is at some level similar for all the students. We are there focused on the poses, breathing—we are in the moment for the most part. The students are focused, unplugged—there is no talking. It is always quiet; it is still.

The next class, a body-weight flow workout with the fitness center instructor, was an interesting experience for us as participants and frustrating for Kim. In the past, Kim partnered with the previous instructor to introduce students to this type of circuit activity using body weight and movement flow. In past years, the focus was on proper alignment, appropriate movement for body types, and breathing through the exercise sequences. The previous instructor promoted a more holistic approach to resistance training that could be incorporated into anyone's lifestyle and had students pay attention to how they felt before, during, and after movement activities. The new instructor had a different background—she was a competitive weight lifter and a strength/ conditioning coach. She was very knowledgeable, skilled, and had a passion for what she does. She was hired to work with the elite athletes and high-performance teams and is very good at designing training programs for the student-athlete. For the majority of students in our schools, however, introducing them to power exercises with medicine balls and push-up repetitions is not necessarily promoting how to put together a body-weight flow sequence that could be done at home, on the road, in a dorm room, or in the backyard.

The frustration for Kim was twofold: the lack of connection to wellness and holistic health, and how difficult it can be to find instructors who can adapt to teaching in large groups of teenagers. There was a significant amount of standing around as there was only one medicine ball for every five students and without adequate demonstration and explanation of the activities, the students (and I) were unsure what we were supposed to be doing. There is a difference between instruction and teaching. Teaching involves being a teacher, understanding the needs of your students, and planning/responding accordingly. Instruction is more prescriptive, mechanical, and one-size-fits-all. So when you plan for a holistic way of teaching physical education, it includes finding guests who understand a balanced holistic approach and guiding them through how to prepare for teaching a group of adolescents in a school setting.

Our first belly-dancing class began with choosing a hip scarf. I must admit even I was eager to put one on to hear it shake and create its own music from body movement. The energy in the room was nervous excitement and Kim reminded us that we needed to focus, bring some calmness in the room, pay attention to ourselves, and "get in tune" with our bodies. Our warmup consisted of breathing with simple movement patterns with our hips, legs, and arms. Done slowly, these movements were actually a type of dynamic stretching. It is an odd feeling to move your hips, arms, and legs in this way as much of our body movement in physical education does not promote movement along all planes at the same time. This "unlocking" of the core, hips, and pelvis is also key to a healthy lifestyle and injury prevention because the dominant posture patterns in modern society involve forward flexion in a static sitting position. I noticed immediately that my hips were just not going to move the way I was asking them and realized how locked everything was.

The next class, Olympian Georgette Reed[1] came to speak to the students. While her background was competitive sport at an elite level, her message when she recounted the story of her athlete experiences emphasized "balance" and the importance of paying attention to the emotional and spiritual dimensions of the self. She talked about how not listening to our bodies can result in overtraining and injury, as it did for her. She learned over the years that while sometimes it is very difficult to navigate through the opinions of others, media messaging, or peer pressure, you have to find your own way to move and find a balance. You have to learn to live for now, and be willing to adapt and trust in each path that life takes you on. Georgette further explained,

A lot of times in life you make plans, which is great. But sometimes a wrench gets thrown in it and you have to go along a different path. Don't panic, just go with it. Take it in the moment and work with what's happening right here, right now.

She shared that she tries not to label or judge anything as right or wrong, good or bad; it just is.

Use whatever happens as an opportunity. Keep shining; enjoy every second of every day. Keep moving. I believe—love myself and I'm going to do my best to share me with others. Be as genuine, creative, and unique an individual as you can be.

Students were completely engaged in this class. Georgette had captured their attention, and her caring demeanor filled the room with a supportive energy. She told the class that best thing they can do is believe in themselves and the next best thing is to believe in others and give to others. She was open to questions and dialogue, and encouraged discussion. It was a great example of how curriculum comes to life by reaching into the community to bring meaningful conversation about the journey of life from multiple perspectives. This is an active, dynamic curriculum that extends beyond the walls of the classroom.

I found the beginning of the next class particularly noteworthy, as it was a good example of how Kim was not afraid of showing vulnerability. Students were able to hear about Kim's struggles with illness and pain. She told the story about her weekend driving the volleyball team in the school bus to an out-of-town tournament. It was incredibly stressful and she woke up at 4:00 a.m. with an intense migraine headache. She could not move and it brought her to tears. In years past, she would have turned to painkillers but now she uses yoga, meditation, and relaxation. This is what she did that night and she felt better. She explained how she had to recognize the source of her stress and address it with mindful practice. She emphasized, however, that sometimes it may be necessary to incorporate Western medicine. After several days of her own practice and listening to her body, it was evident that she was faced with something beyond just stress. She promptly went to the local Medicentre and confirmed her suspicion that she had an ear infection.

I understood why she felt this was important to share. Many students in the room do not have a chance to dialogue about health issues and mainstream messaging supports a pharmaceutical approach where students are popping pills more and more. Kim wanted students to know that there are alternatives and that the best way to deal with things is to understand the source of your stress and address that. Being mindful of our day-to-day activities and how our body feels acts as a barometer for our own health in the future. Connecting body, mind, and spirit allows us to be proactive, not reactive to many health issues.

The following week's observation and participation included two very different activities: a classroom lecture on the topic of training principles and a Moksha yoga class. It was very interesting to participate in the lecture as one of the students. I paired up with another girl and we shared a booklet to follow along with Kim's lesson. There was no question that Kim made the information as interesting and relevant as she could for us. She used many personal stories, connected into Georgette Reed's discussion, and gave practical examples that would relate to the life-worlds of the students. Students followed the PowerPoint presentation as the slides reviewed basic components of fitness—strength/power, endurance, cardiovascular fitness, flexibility, and body composition, as well as training principles (FITT, specificity, progressive overload, etc.) and energy systems (aerobic, anaerobic-lactic, anaerobic-alactic). As the information became more technical, I could feel myself drifting. We were asked to discuss the difference between isokinetic, isometric, and isotonic. I thought I remembered but was not confident, so my partner and I Googled it. What I realized then is how different it is now from when I was in school or even five years ago as a teacher. Information is at our students' fingertips and now more than ever I question the usefulness of lecture-type lessons in physical and health education. It is doubtful that understanding the level of detail that was incorporated into this required, department-prescribed PowerPoint would result in students applying the information to their own lives. Students need to be active with these principles, with the epistemological knowledge being the byproduct. So what Kim did was brilliant, she repeated a key theme throughout—balance. Instead of just talking about ratio of strength, endurance, cardiovascular workouts per week, she simplified it and reminded us about the principle of balance. She reminded us about the balance of activities we do in the course and how it is not just one type of exercise. Balance also applies to nutrition, water intake, sleep, social life, etc. Learning how to live a healthy life is not about understanding terms on a page; it is about how we incorporate balance in our lives. That will be different for everyone and requires listening to our bodies. Kim cautions students about all the different training programs and diets that are advertised, and the unrealistic female body type that is portrayed in the media.

> Be happy with the body you have. I don't want you to "diet"—I want you to eat healthy. Go to belly-dance class, walk the dog, meet your friends for a hike, join a team—it's about a balanced lifestyle, not fad programs or diets.

For these students, healthy living is more about being able to scrutinize and question all the fitness, diet, and health fads that the market-driven economy feeds our children and youth. We need to guide them in how to access reliable and accurate information that can help them live healthfully. We need to encourage them to question if what they are seeing, hearing, experiencing is balanced—socially, emotionally, spiritually, physically.

For several weeks, Kim prepared us for the Moksha yoga class. The day of the class, we all arrived with our gear—three towels, water bottle, sweat-band or bandana for hair, and a change of clothes. I was nervous and so were many of the girls. Here I was, an adult, more than 10 years teaching physical education, an ex-athlete who has done countless types of workouts, and I was nervous going into a yoga studio that I had never been to before. As soon as I walked into the room, the intensity of the heat and humidity hit me hard. I set up my mat and towel, positioned my water bottle, and lay down. I focused on my breathing as Kim suggested, and not the elephant-on-my-chest feeling that I was experiencing. It was hot and I was already sweating immensely. The instructor started the class and I followed her instructions. Many times I misinterpreted what she said but Kim warned us that this may happen and to just keep focused on breathing and adjust on the next pose. It was slippery and—the only other word that really fits—icky. Sweat dripped off my earlobes and nose, ran into my ears, down my back, chest, buttocks, legs, between my toes. It was hard to not stop every second to wipe myself off with a towel. I kept going back to my breathing—long, strong breaths in, audible exhalations. I lost my grip on the mat/towel several times and had to readjust and keep breathing. Many times I stopped and went into child's pose to regroup and focus. Finally we got to the end and went into Savasana and were allowed to stay as long as we wanted. I wiped off the excess sweat and lay down—only to find the sweat continuing to pour out of my pores.

The following week I participated in a belly-dance class and attended a session on Reiki with a guest instructor from the community. At the beginning of the belly-dance class, Kim explained why she was absent from class the previous day. She talked about how she had to stop and listen to her body, how she did not always do that in the past and her health suffered. She also told students about her mother who never took a day off as a teacher/principal and now in retirement, her body has literally collapsed. It is cumulative, Kim explained, and then asked, "How many of you know when you are getting sick? Do you ignore or listen to the signs? What do you do? How did you get there?" She discussed the issue further by recommending a book titled *When the Body Says No* by Dr. Gabor Maté. When you constantly say yes and give your energy away, your body will say no for you in the form of ill health. It is important to listen to your body, recognize what your own signs are, and understand the role that hidden stress can play in your overall health.

We began the belly-dance class with a warmup using the same key principles of yoga—focus, breath, and feel your body. During class, Kim reminded us to relax, feel the music, feel the beat, and enjoy. "Don't worry if you're not quite getting it," she said, "we have lots of time." The class was preparing for a performance that was to take place during the opening ceremonies of one of the city's premier basketball tournaments. The routine was coming along and Kim was mostly working with students on refinement. All the students were engaged—there was a feeling of excitement, laughter, smiling, giggling but focused. Everyone was present and the atmosphere was light. This was an environment where students can take risks. I overheard one student say it is the only class where she can "make a fool of herself" and "it doesn't matter if you make a mistake, you're still okay." The cool down was quiet and I was surprised how quickly the energy became so calm. We moved into a stretch (runner's lunge) and there was some grunts, groans, and giggles—Kim swiftly but gently brought them back to their breath and focus. We finished with child's pose and then a hug—"give yourself a hug, you did great today! You are all awesome!"

The class on Reiki was interesting and captured our attention regarding energy and the body. The instructor explained that *rei* means "universal energy" and *ki* (Japanese form of Qi) means "individual life-force/energy." He emphasized that Reiki is spiritual and not anything to do with a religion. It is based on values to promote harmony and peace within ourselves and among each other. The basic premise of Reiki is the transfer of universal energy through the hands to re-establish normal flow of *ki*, which then can promote the natural ability of the body to heal. The instructor led us through some activities to experience feeling energy and exercises using Reiki energy. One particular activity I felt was important, especially for teenagers, was understanding that energy transfer requires a "good connection," which means that we have to be open to receive; we have to listen. If we are disconnected, everyone will be trying to talk, but if we are connected, the energy will flow to the next person.

The most significant part of the next class was the return of a previous H2O student. She now teaches hip-hop in the community and is taking courses at the local college. She wanted to give back and gain experience teaching dance in the school setting. As with many of the other guest instructors, she quickly realized that teaching teenagers in a school is very different from teaching a community or college recreation class. Her breakdown of the hip-hop dance into simpler moves was going well until she tried to add music. At this point, she lost most of us because the music was too fast. The fascinating part is some of the girls were really quite good, and others, like me, were awkward. But it did not seem to matter—we all just laughed, enjoyed ourselves, and accepted the fact that we were going to bump into one another. Some of the moves we did were supposed to have "attitude" and the girls had a good laugh at my attempt, which resembled more of a Halloween zombie than a hip-hop dancer. It speaks to the atmosphere in the class and the level of comfort students began to have with their own bodies—moving in ways that we are not used to. It provides a body awareness that other activities do not have. We moved in so many different planes and directions, utilizing muscles I'm sure some did not know they had. At the end of class, Kim wanted us to pay attention to

> how good it feels to have your body move! Feel your heart beating, the energy. Pay attention to how we were in class—we laughed, we moved, we sweated—and the break we got from the stressors of our day to just enjoy the class.

As we finished the class with some yoga stretching, Kim talked about how she hoped that they could find a place for what they learned today—"whether it is at a wedding, a social dance, function at university, a class—maybe you'll remember what we did and participate."

The last class in October, Halloween day, H2O students joined their Community Learning Skills program (CLS) buddies to play a game of "minute to win it." This was a great activity for both groups. For the CLS students, being involved in a game is a big accomplishment, and the H2O students supported their buddies to participate in a challenge. Standing up to try something new is a big risk for many of the students from both classes. The room was loud with cheering, and full of energy as students took turns with different activities. We finished early and went back to the H2O studio to debrief. The class agreed that everyone was smiling and the energy was incredibly positive, even from those who did not participate in a challenge. Kim mentioned that this positive energy is the reason we do these things.

> We want to surround ourselves with positive people every day. So you want to pay attention and think about the people around you—think about the feeling and the energy in that room where we just were and use it as your guide when you make choices of who you want to have in your life.

Kim finished this class with a review of what their report cards would look like this year for this course, as they were being distributed next week. She reviewed how the intent of the class is about how you treat yourself and others every day, outside and inside of class. On paper, what this looks like is not only their participation in class activities, but volunteering, participation with the Community Learning Skills, being prepared for class, engagement with guest speakers/instructors, leadership activities, and fitness testing. Kim then remarked,

> But please remember what I want for you in this course. Lifelong health habits—you don't have to run on the treadmill at a gym to be healthy. You can walk, do yoga, line dance, or do your own circuit. And be nice to yourself and others—that's difficult to mark in a traditional setting but you need to know you're all doing great. You come to class, participate, and every day you leave smiling. You can't really put a value on holistic health. You have to be kind to yourself and each other. This is what I want you to take with you.

The first week of November was very characteristic of a school week during a major winter storm in Alberta. With two snow days and Kim away for a volleyball tournament, attendance was quite low in class. In addition to yoga on Monday, Kim introduced foam rollers to students. I reflected on Kim's words at the end of yoga class and wondered how many of us, as teachers, encourage this type of connection:

> Feel your body as it thanks you for slowing down and taking the time to take care of yourself this morning. Hands on your chest, feel your heart beating, the energy in your fingertips, feel your blood pulsing through your veins/body. Thank you for being here today.

Rollers are firm foam cylinders that are primarily used for tissue massage and are a good alternative to a formal massage therapy. Kim explains it to students in this way: "Sometimes it's like there are cobwebs over your muscles, or knots, so you want to smooth this out, keep moving and rolling helps clear things." The rollers we used were homemade from PVC pipe wrapped in yoga mat material.

Rolling can sometimes be painful, as we all soon discovered. Again, Kim reminded the class to be as mindful and as present as possible. You want to pay attention to your muscle, and much like when you are at the massage therapist, you want to breathe through it and relax (avoid talking). She put on some relaxing music and led us through the technique of rolling, starting with the calf muscles and working our way up the body. After we finished, she encouraged students to assess how they feel after every workout and take the time to notice whether they feel relaxed, sore, calm, or something else.

> As life gets busy, take the time to take care of yourself—take the time to relax. Rollers are an easy way to relieve some tension…and cheaper than a $100 massage! When you're sitting in front of the TV, use the roller and your body will thank you.

Kim developed the next lesson to show students how to navigate through the onslaught of health information that is constantly bombarding the public. She emphasized that she is not an expert but wants to raise awareness of a few issues and some misinformation that is present in the media, as well as how to become an informed consumer. Students brainstormed about nutritional information in the media and discussed how you never see a commercial about eating an apple or anything healthy. Kim highlighted how the majority of food advertised on TV should be avoided because it is mostly processed, high in sodium, preservatives, and other additives. Other nutrition topics included genetically modified organisms (GMO), pesticide use, and organic food labeling. I think this was a refreshing alternative to the traditional "four food groups" lesson most nutrition classes cover.

Students were also asked to bring a personal care (e.g., cosmetic, shampoo, perfume) container they use on a regular basis. Kim then presented a list similar to the "Dirty Dozen" ingredient list published by the David Suzuki Foundation (2010). This research identifies that "one in eight of the 82,000 ingredients used in personal care products are industrial chemicals, including carcinogens, pesticides, reproductive toxins, and hormone disruptors." Students used the list to scrutinize the products that they are currently using and discuss alternatives. This led to the discussion of why students felt they needed to use makeup or perfume. While there were a variety of responses, the common theme was about body image. Kim then showed a video titled, "11 facts about body image" and opened a dialogue about loving the body we have. This all tied back into the concept of balance that they had previously discussed during the lesson on training principles. I was impressed by their understanding of the complexities of the issues, willingness to consider other ideas and alternatives, and desire to connect this information and dialogue to not only their own emotional, physical, spiritual health, but the health of the planet as well.

As their Middle Eastern dance performance was drawing near, Kim moved the students to practice in a gymnasium setting. On this day I was strictly an observer, as they needed to practice with the formations and numbers they would have for the final performance. Because I had been a participant in the class for the most part, students were comfortable with me watching, and even asked for my feedback. It was interesting to watch them, knowing where they started ten weeks before.

One H2O student who was not feeling well sat down beside me and she remarked about how great she thought belly dancing is and that *everyone* should try it. She believes it is a good stress release (mental break), a good ab-dominal exercise, and whole body workout. It is fun—a distraction where you just focus on the dance and the music is great. The conversation continued as we watched the class prepare. She asked me about my research and then commented about how difficult it was to focus on taking care of ourselves (body–mind–spirit). As I was observing and recording field notes on this day, I was able to write down some of her comments.

> It's just so busy. I'm not sure how we slow down the world. I think the adults need to help too. It's kind of like they set the pace. We can point it out to them but…it's just frustrating.

Kim was now in the refining phase of instruction, fine-tuning, positioning, and timing. She was using humor to distract students from the repetition of practice. The group was really coming together, not just with the dance it-self but also as a supportive community. The students were encouraging each other, their bodies and energy moving synchronically. At the end of class, we shifted to the large gym where the actual performance would take place. There were two other classes sitting in stands after changing, which caused some nervous reluctance to practice. Kim assured them that they could do this and reminded them how great they are, regardless of who is watching. Furthermore, the following week would be in front of a packed house, so trying it out today with 60 people watching would be a good start. They performed the dance well and were surprised when the audience clapped and cheered. It was impressive and I think the teachers and students were surprised that there was a class in the school that was able to prepare something so different and complex. It was a great confidence booster for the H2O students.

The following week I arrived at the gym early in preparation for the open-ing ceremonies and belly-dance performance. The students were very nervous and asked if I would help them with the music, to do one quick practice before the stands began to fill. We then went to the section of the stands desig-nated for performers and watched the ceremonies begin. This tournament is a long-standing tradition in the school with a number of girls' and boys' teams from Western Canada. Kim's attempt to expose people to different activities happening in the physical education department into a decades-old tradi-tional sporting event is to be admired. As I watched the H2O class perform on the gym floor that would soon be host to several intense basketball games, I realized how much courage and confidence it took for the students to dance in front of hundreds of peers, parents, community members, and guests. I also thought about how each dancer was sharing this experience with the community. Kim introduced it well and highlighted the connections to holistic health. A boy sitting beside me who was waiting to perform with his break-dancing group commented on how good the class was and how important it was for them to perform at this event. "We need more of this, more options. People need to see that there's more out there than just this [pointing to the basketball]." This is part of Kim's vision—to expose people to culture, to contribute to our communities, to think differently about movement and health, and to achieve balance in our lives.

After this activity, Kim and I decided that I had spent enough time observing the class, and with the winter holidays approaching, scheduling would be somewhat repetitive. What was needed now was to make some final decisions on how we would articulate what it means to teach a wellness-oriented physical education curriculum.

Circling Back to Stillness: Synthesis

A journey toward stillness where one is "available, individually or collectively, for deeper insight into what the present moment holds." (Smith, 1999, p. 4)

This journey began with the process of *currere* and an understanding of curriculum as *currere*. Recall that *currere* is the Latin infinitive understanding of curriculum meaning the "running of the course." It refers back to Roman chariot races. Metaphorically, this is an important part of our inquiry because this journey track is circular in nature—we started this active curriculum inquiry and came back to a "home base" in a new way. This is much the same as the circling back in the synthesis stage of *currere*, going from the wholeness of the present, paying attention to the progressive and regressive, then understanding how the pieces of the past and future are part of the "new" present moment.

I work to get a handle on what I've been and what I imagine myself to be, so I can wield this information, rather than it wielding me. The beginning of agency. Now the antithesis, the synthetical stage. More deeply, now, in the present. I choose what of it to honor, what of it to let go. I choose again who it is I aspire to be, how I wish my life history to read. I determine my social commitments; I devise my strategies: whom to work with, for what, and how. (Pinar & Grumet, 1976, p. ix)

> Make it all a whole. It, all of it—intellect, emotion, behavior—occurs in and through the physical body. As the body is a concrete whole, so what occurs within and through the body can become a discernible whole, integrated in its meaningfulness... Mind in its place, I conceptualize the present situation, I am placed together. Synthesis. (Pinar & Grumet, 1976, p. 61)

It may appear that the stages of *currere* were done in a linear fashion; however, this was not the case. While there was a chronological nature to our discussions, there is simultaneity in understanding the past and future in the present moment along the way. In other words, at any point in the semester, there were times that we would bring together the past, present, and future, and this gave us greater knowledge of the present moment. Progressive and regressive experiences that surfaced as we moved through the weeks were added to ones previously identified and an ongoing analysis of their relationality to each other took place. Although we often stepped into synthesizing what all of these parts meant, many times throughout the semester, we were careful to leave those thoughts suspended in a metaphysical "space" so that they may, if needed, become bracketed again. It allowed the question to remain open until we were able to find a still point for synthesis.

The synthetical stage of *currere* is a time of stillness, a meditative practice that we are able to take all the pieces of our self—intellectual, physical, emotional, and spiritual, make it all whole and re-enter a more meaningful present. It was a time to focus on understanding the world that was still unfolding in front of us, without getting lost in it. We reviewed and discussed all our writings, the regressive, progressive, the analytical and our synthetical moments throughout the semester to come to some conclusions about how certain aspects contribute to what it means to *be* a teacher of holistic health, what it means to teach a wellness approach in physical education. We view that there is no separation between personal–professional, body–mind, mother–wife–teacher, student–researcher, class–life-world, and as such this "coming home" stage, the pedagogical moment of synthesis, presented enlightenment moments about ourselves as human beings connected to others, to the world.

The next chapter will present what we came to understand about what it means to teach a wellness-oriented physical education curriculum. However, what is not included in that chapter is how the process of co-constructing this meaning impacted our individual identities and ways of being. The following section will show some of Kim's synthetical moments, "rewritten" present about who she is and becoming as a (w)holistic being. In addition, I share some of my own synthetical musings about who I am and becoming as an individual connected to the greater cosmos.

Kim: Being and Becoming

One of the most significant synthesis moments for Kim was revisiting a traumatic car accident and teaching event in her past, and the experiences related to those events. These continued to be a source of pain for her and had negatively affected her emotional, physical, and spiritual wellbeing. Gradually, she identified specific regressive events, experiences, and key people that all fed into these traumatic events. She also described progressive ideas that represented future possibilities. In stillness, she could name these events and experiences and begin to let them flow back into the energy of the universe, a process of letting go. Through this process, we were able to see the contribution of these moments to who she is as a whole being and how who she is as a whole provided a meaningful (re)conceptualization of the present situation.

> So this one was hard again. The story I wasn't happy with...obviously it was the car accident and everything. So hitting rock bottom...Coaching, the pressure.... I don't know what else would've made me quit coaching. I would never on my own because there's always another student—there's a great grade-9 girl coming up or it's their grade-12 year, then it goes on. They would've never let me quit. The girls would have kept saying, "oh, just one more year" and I would still be coaching today. So hitting rock bottom...what else would have worked, nothing else would have worked. I'm sure I would've been in another bad relationship and coaching weekends and evenings, no life.

> That pressure...was so overwhelming and then to have such a public mistake...and to be able to forgive myself for that has been very difficult because it seems like that was a different person. I do believe now I have forgiven myself...you have to let it go...look what happened to you when you didn't look after yourself and realizing now through this...understanding the holistic picture.... So I just think I can look back on all of that now and then look at [new husband] and I look at the life I have and the studio and baby and I have to say thank you that that happened to me. So the universe led me in another direction that I am grateful for. I am the happiest I have ever been—I'm going to start to cry. This has been so emotional for me. This was so very powerful. So, yeah, just putting it in a different lens—that was really interesting to do that.

Kim's rewriting of this event incorporated her vision for the future—for herself, her family, and her students. Her belief that taking care of the self (and by doing so, others)—emotionally, spiritually, physically, mentally—illustrates more clearly her way of living, who she is as a person, and consequently how she teaches.

Kim explained how she originally thought that the impetus for starting this course was completely selfish. At the time, she was dissatisfied with her career.

> I knew I liked teaching, but I didn't like the environment I was in or the structure, so I just created my own [course].

But as we discussed more regressive and progressive events throughout the semester, she began to place these into a relational theme. The negative teaching environment was not the only factor in her designing this course; it was her own health, to be a better teacher and consequently a concern for students' health.

> So looking after myself, my health…starting the yoga, the belly-dance classes, and just doing stuff for myself. And because I am a teacher and I like to share, I wanted to teach my students how to do this. Oh my God, if I would have learned this 20 years ago!… So it was for me to be a better teacher, for me to enjoy what I was teaching…and I saw the need with the students today….and now it has just taken on a life of its own and has grown.

Kim also talked about who/where she wanted to be in the future.

> I want to ensure this program continues to grow in this school. I want H2O to be its own course somehow someday. They just have to catch up with us so we will wait for them to catch up with us. Now I have the confidence and if I could go with you to HPEC and GETCA [conferences].… I want to go there to actually pass on knowledge.

When talking about her new understandings from this journey about teaching a wellness-oriented approach, Kim explained,

> For me in August, yoga was mindfulness and now all activities are mindful. So just carrying that broader spectrum. In August, I was upset that students weren't always getting it, some skipping class and stuff. I'm more patient now and they will realize someday the benefits and you helped me reinforce that. Again I believed that but to talk to somebody else was good. And I was uncertain about the future of H2O and now the press, the interest, it's going full-steam ahead. In August, I was just happy having this program and keeping it quiet, and now I'm more determined to expand it.

> And then, of course, just how I've grown, the reflection, how I've changed parts of the course…because I had kind of plateaued and was looking for ideas. I was like a sponge with all these guest speakers coming in but they just would talk on their small little areas, whereas

you came in with the umbrella, a blanket of that could cover this whole course. And that's what I feel we've done—it wasn't just "fix this and fix that." It's like, "let's tie everything we are doing together." In August, it was we do this on this day, that on that day, and it was a whole bunch of different little programs. I was running a Phys. Ed. class with a holistic class, and now it is one holistic class.

In the end, we discussed what Kim thought about the future and her way of being, and how she would tell a new story for herself—teacher of H2O, mother-to-be, all of it.

Honestly I think it's about being in the moment—I want to enjoy every moment. I'm much more grateful and I just have this calm about being here and what will happen will happen. I'm not scared about parenting at all. I'm not scared about being a wife and mother. I'm not scared about where this course is going to go…. This movement is happening even without me, so it's going. And the press have been great; there's already a buzz that is happening so…I'm hoping that even in two or three years, it's not just about me…if other teachers are now teaching it in the city…. Like I said, it is all bigger than me. Some people think that I am so possessive and that I don't want anyone else teaching this. No, I wouldn't have given it away if I am perfectly healthy and happy to teach it, but if other people can teach it and do a good job, then I'm happy.

Michelle: Being and Becoming

For me, there were many synthetical moments on this journey that have influenced my way of being and who I am becoming as an individual connected to the greater cosmos. How I wrote the previous statement is a testament to how I now look at "research" and who I am/becoming. Prior to this inquiry, I would have compartmentalized, fragmented myself as a scholar and focused on developing the researcher, as if who I was outside of the academic environment had little influence. Living and breathing a curriculum of wellness requires the whole self.

I learned that stillness is a requirement for me to be a healthy person, and as such, participate fully in the world—inquiry project, home, classroom, forest, community, gymnasium, meeting room, or river valley path. Mindfulness became central to our project, just as it is in our lives. When you practice in this way, you can sense the interconnectedness among all living things, and as such, all the qualitative-research-recommended "techniques" for authentic conversations, building/maintaining collaborative relationships, mediating power dynamics, for example, are no longer technical research skills to master, they are part of the ethic of participating in the inquiry process. Mindful awareness means that you name the dilemmas that may be unfolding, which equates to what others may refer to as the researcher maintaining objectivity.

The reflectiveness and reflexiveness of this wisdom-guided inquiry also meant that I had to be willing to let go of what I knew at the start and be willing to hear others' points of view to be able to move in a more creative manner (Winter, 2003). I learned how to truly listen with my real attention—"abandon[ing] or put[ting] aside all prejudices, preformulations and daily activities" (Krishnamurti, 1954, as cited in Kumar, 2013, p. 91). To help with the concept of nonpermanence, Kim and I agreed on the use of a "critical friend" to gain different perspectives on the process. The concept of a critical friend comes from action research literature and is described as "someone who would be a support and act as a sounding board...help the action researcher address dilemmas that may arise" (Stenhouse, 1975). Herr and Anderson (2005) believe that having several critical friends allows for a range of different responses to the work and ensures bias and subjectivity are critically examined and not ignored (Lomax, Woodward & Parker, as cited in Herr & Anderson, 2005). Responses I received from the critical friends were brought forward into the discussions with Kim so that everything remained transparent in the co-researcher relationship.

While action research was not the only process we relied upon to help inform us in this wisdom-guided inquiry, it was an integral part. After living this process, when it comes to evaluating quality, I would agree with Herr and Anderson's (2005) claim that the terms *validity* or *trustworthiness* are not appropriate in wisdom-guided inquiry because neither acknowledges its action-oriented outcomes. The authors explain that "action researchers, like all researchers, are interested in whether knowledge generated from the research is valid or trustworthy, but they are usually also interested in outcomes that go beyond knowledge generation" (p. 49). In addition, the autobiographical roots of the *currere* process have a transformatory nature to be able to gain insight at a deeper more humanistic level where teachers, in tracing the origins of their educational experience, co-construct meaning in relationship to the Other, and to the world. Britzman (1991) reminds us of the significance of conducting research with teachers in this way:

> First, images of theory as reflective practice can dissipate a view of theory as imposed from above and situate it as constructed rather than received. Second, in positioning theory as dialogic to lived experience, the traditional dualism of theory and practice can be reconceptualized as a problem of praxis. When this occurs, practice can

be understood theoretically. Third, an emphasis on personal practical knowledge values the activity of theorizing as a tenuous yet transformative activity. Teachers can experience themselves as authors and interpreters of their lived experience. To see teachers as interpreters of theory dismantles the view of theory as monological. Finally, these research directions re-establish a qualitative understanding of the complexities of teachers' work. Through the use of qualitative research methods, research grounded in the voices and in the contradictory realities of teachers implicitly opposes technocratic research directions that seek to "improve" education without the teachers' knowledge. (p. 54)

Prior to this journey, I was concerned about the general research community's reaction to our "method" and acceptance of the knowledge we would share. In the past, I have been surrounded by systems and people who tend to solely value empirical practices and epistemological ways of knowing. My experiences being a co-researcher with Kim reinforce my views on how important this type of inquiry is to reconnecting, restoring, and reviving the health of our students, institutions, communities, and the planet. It gives the statistics a voice, a spirit. While there may still be those who are critical of the objectivity of the researcher, I contest that the lack of subjectivity in research is a big part of why we continue to perpetuate the status quo.

As I made final edits to this chapter, some time had passed since this particular moment of synthesis. Recently Kim and I had the opportunity to present our story about her class to teachers, scholars, and community members at a national physical and health education conference in Canada. Leading up to the conference, Kim expressed concern about no one showing up to our session. Reinforcing my views on the value of this type of inquiry and perspective, our session was standing-room only, with people spilling out into the hallway trying to catch as much of our presentation as possible. The sincere interest and desire to learn about a different way of looking at physical education curriculum and inquiry was clearly evident in that room that day.

· 5 ·

TEACHING A
CURRICULUM OF WELLNESS
IN PHYSICAL EDUCATION

Curriculum is breathing, living, moving
Ongoing, practicing, interconnected being, a way
My spirit just knows at a level I cannot describe
My body pays full attention to the spirit to be well
My mind is guided by the spirit and body in simultaneous flow
Spirit, body, mind—synergy, balance, energy flowing
Disrupted and betrayed when put into text.
— MICHELLE KILBORN

As I considered how to present the insights we gained, I was at odds with how to capture in text *the way* this teacher was in her ongoing practice of teaching adolescents to live healthfully in the world. How she is as a teacher connects to her philosophical beliefs of kind, compassionate living in balance and wellness. *How* she teaches is who she is. She does not just pass on knowledge to students in hopes they are listening; she lives curriculum with them. This journey of practicing a life of wellness that she shares with her students goes beyond following a set of learning outcomes or performance standards. It is an emotional, spiritual, mental, and physical journey—a dynamic, open, and active process of living in a moral disposition that encourages nonperfection, nonpermanence, and nonduality. This is a way of being, not an act of performance.

It cannot be represented in a model, distributed in a handout with a to-do checklist, developed into a program, or designed into a ready-made kit.

If I were to follow my technocratic tendencies from the past, I would have organized what we learned together in a nice, neat report with definitive themes and categories with clear-cut distinguishing characteristics. However, this would misrepresent the nature of what it means to teach in this way. What we lived in that semester was messy—there were many events, experiences, ideas, and moments of enlightenment that are dynamically intertwined within the energy of body, mind, spirit, and heart of individuals and the energy of the Earth and cosmos. The dynamic, active, flowing nature of learning how to be healthy and well cannot be titrated into an epistemological formula that consists of fragmented parts. It needs to be whole.

The following chapter characterizes how Kim participates in a curriculum of wellness with her students and attempts to portray *the way* a teacher is with her students to help them learn how to live holistically, how to live well. There are eleven "pedagogical moments" that emerged from our analysis: journey of life; this is not a kit; mindfulness; feeling confident; interconnectedness: kindness and connecting beyond the self; building community; communicating and sharing stories; balance; to test or not to test: merging poles; (non)assessment of wellness; and Holistic Health Option (H2O) as the new HPE. Of course, there is a situatedness to these pedagogical moments that I sometimes attempt to explain further, and other times, I let Kim's voice/writing speak for itself.

It should be noted that the headings serve more as an organizing strategy; but similar to the concern that Armour (2006) raises, I am aware that in doing this I may be undermining my desire to represent wholeness and interconnectedness, as these sections appear as fragmented, disconnected themes. As such, I encourage readers to weave the following writings with the text of the inquiry journey stories you have already experienced in previous chapters.

Journey of Life

A key piece to teaching a curriculum of wellness in physical education is the reconceptualization of curriculum. Throughout the semester, it was evident that this way of teaching was dependent upon Kim's nontraditional perspective of curriculum. Her way of thinking about curriculum was more about the journey of life for the students and herself:

There is no endpoint for H2O.... What are you going to do February 1st when you start school and you have no Phys. Ed.? What are you going to do February to June to stay healthy and mindful, active and fit—that's an issue and this class is not over in January. This will be a practice for the rest of their life, and habits for the rest of their life. So that ties into the 80 minutes a day. But it also ties into it's not over in January and they need to hopefully absorb what we're doing

This isn't an 80-minute class everyday—it's 24 hours a day, seven days a week—how you're living, what you're thinking, what you're putting into your body and what's coming out of your body, your activities, your happiness. That's what this course is about—it's about your journey, your lifestyle.

This life journey philosophy has a significant impact on how Kim is as a teacher and her decision making in what she does with students. She looks at her own life journey and incorporates some of her learning experiences into her programming.

Nothing I did in Phys. Ed [as a student] I do now.... I can't play basketball; I can't do a lot of things. I still swim and I guess I run but in this class, these are all activities that they can continue to do. Especially when we did the circuit I explained to them I did this circuit all last summer—I did Tabata at the cabin. You don't need a fancy gym membership and you can belly dance at home. It's a lifestyle approach. Just giving them all the options. Even when we go over to the elementary school—we're walking over there.

This Is Not a Kit

Throughout the semester Kim spoke of requests from other schools to send them her course. It seems they wanted the quick-and-easy binder filled with ready-made lesson plans and a kit of equipment to go with it. She explained to them that there really was not a magic formula or checklist; it is multifaceted:

It's not so much "how well you perform the activities" but rather "how does it *feel* when you are performing these activities." We have guest speakers, we volunteer in the community, and our entire course is based around mindfulness.

Consistently, inquiring teachers would only look at the sample list of activities that Kim would give as examples and miss the messaging about the course being more about *how* you teach the activities, rather than *what* you teach. Even though she explained that you choose the activities based on minimal equipment, community partnerships, and mindful practice, they persisted with requests for a prescriptive method. The learning outcomes are facilitated through action and doing, and are not attached to any specific physical activity but primarily activities you could do for life. Furthermore, the way students participate should support their own wellness and that of the community and the planet.

> It is not content focused, it is process…

> It is more about the process, or their [students'] progress over the content. You know our belly-dancing routine is not going to be perfect and it's going to be all over the place and it's going to be some people moving this way and some people moving that way—when I picture it and all 50 of us out there trying to do it. But that's not the point of it, belly dancing is not meant to be perfect.

Mindfulness

The most prominent principle that grounds Kim's H2O course is mindfulness. Kabat-Zinn (1990) characterizes mindfulness as

> moment-to-moment awareness. It is cultivated by purposefully paying attention to things we ordinarily never give a moment's thought to. It is a systematic approach to developing new kinds of control and wisdom in our lives, based on our inner capacities for relaxation, paying attention, awareness, and insight. (p. 2)

Kim encourages the cultivation of mindfulness among her students through role modeling, storytelling, discussion, community service, and leading mindful practice in a variety of activities (i.e., yoga, dance, circuit training, walking, meditation). One way she refers to this concept with her students is through the acronym WIN: "what's important now." She learned this from a university instructor when she was a student and it is meant to remind us to stop and pay attention to what is important in this moment, now. She reminds students that there are many things right in front of us that we can learn from; we just have to pay attention. To guide students and help them understand what she means by "paying attention," it is not uncommon for Kim to stop the class to explain her awareness in the moment. For example, while leading the class in yoga, she drew our attention to the fact that she was having difficulty balancing and explained that her thoughts were not here in the classroom—she was preoccupied with the details of a tournament she was organizing. She then returned her focus to her breath, let the thoughts of the tournament pass through, and continued her practice.

Having awareness of our bodies and paying attention to the connection between our body, mind, and spirit is an important part of overall wellness. Kim often refers students back to how their body feels when they are participating in an activity or after they have finished. She believes that so often people do not pay attention to what is really going on in their people bodies, they do not connect into what it feels like when they do something—an anesthetic way of being that is accompanied by disembodied experience (Irwin, 2006).

> So how does this feel? I want you to have the tools to know how good it feels to relax. How good it feels to sweat. Even think back to when we went to Moksha yoga, you were sweating and oh, that felt so good. So just going back and how good did it feel, even after you finished the fitness tests. Were you proud of yourself, how did that feel going to the fitness center, going to run, or working out. So just having them pay attention to their thoughts and feelings when doing stuff. Nothing is accidental, everything has a purpose and everything has a meaning. Why do we work out and if you are just working out to impress somebody else, it doesn't last because that's outside of you. So I think tuning into how good it feels, intrinsic motivation. Even paying attention to eating. So how do you feel after you've eaten a big bag of sugar or how do you feel after you've eaten a really healthy salad…and that's the mindfulness. Just don't sit in front of the TV and eat a bag of chips and just chow down. Chew your food, taste your food.

Irwin (2006) also understands how important it is to "provide experiences that awaken the phenomenological understanding of the balance between, or among, mind, body, emotions, and soul, while providing an experiential approach that may help us make connections between our consciousness and the world around us" (p. 80). This is similar to what Csikszentmihalyi (1997) and Lloyd and Smith (2009) refer to as flow, and considers "how the curricula…may be permeated by a feeling, forming, flowing approach" that focuses "on a qualitative, enlivening engagement of being present with one's body and breath" (p. 3).

Thus, part of mindfulness is paying attention to what is going on in your body while you are active, a type of meditative practice that brackets out the external and promotes real engagement. Too often people disconnect and escape from the experience, which is a type of practice that is then extended to everyday life. This is a key source of our children's increasing levels of physical and mental illness. Smith (2011a) explains, "distractedness, inability to focus and concentrate...increasingly these qualities have come to define the lives of young people" (p. 175). Given the lack of emphasis on meditative sensibilities in contemporary educational institutions, the education system should seriously consider "providing opportunities to teachers and their students to inquire, teach, and learn meditatively and thereby understand and transform their consciousness" (Kumar, 2013, p. 124).

Cultivating mindfulness is a way for youth to begin healing, but as Kim believes, it cannot be forced upon teenagers, it must happen through presenting opportunities for students to see and experience the world in different ways. She does not prescribe what she thinks they should feel or experience; she guides them through a process that allows them to pay attention to their own presence in the human condition. Mindfulness allows us to nourish the body, mind, and spirit and "makes it easier for us to see with greater clarity the way we actually live and therefore how to make changes to enhance our health and the quality of our life" (Kabat-Zinn, 1990, p. 12).

The other side of the principle of mindfulness is Kim's engagement in/with the class. As teachers, it is very easy to get caught up in the day-to-day demands of the job. Kim was incredibly busy—she was the teacher-sponsor for a top provincially ranked high school volleyball team, participated in evening community dance classes in the first trimester of her first pregnancy, coordinated staff social events, organized a provincial basketball tournament, and taught two blocks of social studies and two blocks of the H2O class. Not uncommon to many teachers, this busy schedule makes it difficult to pay attention to the present moment and to be able to notice the pedagogical opportunities. Kim's own mindful practice (and she reminds me that indeed it is about "practicing," as she can get caught up in the swirling chaos of the day-to-day) is a unique aspect of this course. She explains how, as teachers, we have to pay attention to the fact that these are *human beings* in our classrooms and engage with them in a genuine way. This means you have to listen, see, connect—try to understand what is going on in their worlds as teenagers, be able to look into their lives with an open mind, and be willing to accept their way of looking at the world. A simple but powerful example of this mindful practice was Kim paying attention to her students' social lives outside of class. What was in front of her was the fact that Friday is usually "date night." So when you have a physical education class in the afternoon on a Friday, she will not schedule swimming or a high-intensity workout where they would get too sweaty.

> While you may not agree with it, it is their reality, and by scheduling a low-intensity activity such as yoga class on Friday, you get more students showing up and participating.

Aoki (2005) discusses the mindfulness of a situation, "remembering that being in the situation is a human being in his becoming. This mindfulness allows the listening to what it is that a situation is asking" (as cited in Pinar & Irwin, 2005, p. 155). Park (2007) advocates "for the importance of mindfulness as a way of grounding in the immediate daily world of one's self, that of students and the present moment of their intersections" (p. 46). This requires the development of deep listening and a commitment from teachers "to see and work with the reality of students' lives as the curriculum" (Park, 2007, p. 45).

Another example of a mindful way of being is Kim's purposeful scheduling of yoga on Mondays. After the weekend, Kim finds that her students are in desperate need of focus and stillness, a time to unplug. She notes that it is incredibly difficult to find a space or time in school where students can be still. Thus, Kim believes H2O goes "beyond the physicality, beyond physical moving" and creates a space and time for students to be still. This is incredibly important for their overall health.

> So yoga, we always do it Monday to help us let go of the weekend, to focus, let go of your regrets, your fears, everything, start with a clean slate and to go without their cell phones, which is amazing. The Mondays we didn't do yoga, they totally missed it, you missed it. I know that I missed it.

Understanding contemporary youth and what happens when the structure of the school schedule is removed, Kim also addressed the reality of their lives outside of this class.

> So it's not perfect and I tell them…even though you can't do yoga every Monday, what else can you do during that week? Just walk your dog and find a quiet bench? I always try to give them alternatives—if you're on the bus, you can close your eyes on the bus for two minutes in the morning. So even if you're missing your regular routine, you don't want to fall apart. You don't want to become so OCD that if you miss your yoga practice one week you're a disaster. So finding other ways. We did yoga twice in January and both times I said to them while they were waking up—listen to your body, it's asking you to continue to find some quiet space next semester. It's asking you to continue this practice for the rest of your life. So make a promise to yourself that this will not be the last time that you turn off your cell phone. You have to make that a priority.

Feeling Confident

> I want them to feel confident to do stuff on their own, have the confidence to do yoga
> in their basement or out in a class.

A major goal for Kim in this course is for students to have the confidence to continue the activities they are exposed to in class later on in life. To help students to be active on their own, Kim gives them opportunities to lead each other in physical activities that can be done at home with minimal equipment. This is a key factor for high school students, as they will soon be faced with having to take care of themselves without school programing or teacher guidance.

> Next semester especially is when they will realize: wow, I haven't worked out in two
> months. For a lot of them that will be the reality—they will go February to June with-
> out working out.... But if they can go to Gold's gym or they can go to the belly-dance
> studio that's a block away, or Moksha yoga or go for a walk after school a few times
> once a week with a friend. Like I said, just empowering them to have the confidence
> to do that. For me, I was in organized sports so I didn't know anything else. So when
> I could no longer play volleyball and basketball, I was like, hmm, what do I do now?

One strategy she uses to help them build their confidence is a guided process to assist them in being able to perform their own yoga session at home. All of the students become aware of the different categories of the poses and movement patterns (e.g., sitting, kneeling, standing, on stomach and on back), and she simply has them choose one pose from each. After assisting them with this process, the students were amazed that they could do yoga on their own.

> By the end of it they were surprised, "wow, we did it!" And just having the confi-
> dence. I am so big on this...because you want to prepare them for life. You want them
> to have the basics to go out in life, and I just think that this class does that. I'm a very
> confident person and for me to walk into my first yoga class, I was terrified—terrified
> of the skinny, pretty people. Just to give them the confidence to walk into the fitness
> center, to take a Zumba® class...

Students often feel vulnerable going out into the community to participate, and this often leads to avoidance. Kim knows that the key to success is how comfortable students feel going into a new environment and ensuring that they are prepared mentally for the activity. As a participant in the class, I experienced this firsthand when Kim began to talk about going to a Moksha yoga class. I had never been to a hot yoga session and felt very apprehensive about going. For weeks leading up to the field trip, Kim would mention different aspects of what to expect in the class, what we should bring, and what we might feel when we are in the room. She gave examples of what she does to work through the session, how she uses her towels, and warned us that we were going to sweat a great amount. Our discussion following the event highlights the importance of getting students to step outside their comfort zone and preparing them.

Michelle:	As a participant and when you were preparing them [students] and talking about it, I took down those notes because I knew I was going to be trying this out. It was my first time.
Kim:	[surprised] Interesting.
Michelle:	I was nervous. I didn't know what to expect with hot yoga, and you walked us through—bring a beach towel, hand towel, a third towel so that you can shower and change after. Your clothes are going to be soaked, the room temperature, how much water, and I thought, okay, I can do this. And the next time you were telling us…don't worry about it being hard to breathe, and I got in there and I went "holy cow, I don't know if I can do this!" The first 15 minutes was incredibly difficult for me because I'm asthmatic and so I spent a lot of years training myself to try to control my breath, so I know my threshold…a lot of it is mental.
Kim:	It's the panic.
Michelle:	Had you not said all those things ahead of time, I think I would've been in trouble. And the idea that you are absolutely just dripping and it's icky. You said you don't care what they say, that you do wipe your face sometimes, and I thought, okay, she does so I'm going to too. You went through the experience with us and I think that was key.
Kim:	And that's the thing…. You want to prepare your students and set them up for success the best you can, and that's in life, the activities, and everything else. I know when I went to my first Moksha yoga class, I thought I was going to die—the claustrophobia set in and so I know what it's like to go to a first class, so just being able to talk them through it, to tell them about the recovery positions and lead them through and let them know that you're going to be okay. There is enough oxygen in the room and you're not going to boil to death. And I think they knew that.

Not all of the activities that Kim chose to include in the class were always well received by the students. But how Kim approached these situations often resulted in valuable lessons, regardless of how successful students were at executing the activity. For example, many struggled with the Zumba® classes and Kim feared that she was "turning them off" of physical activity. The level of difficulty was high, progressions were very fast, and students were frustrated. However, she managed this situation with encouragement and assurances: "It does not matter if you're not getting all the moves, just keep moving and let's try to have a sense of humor." Because the level of difficulty was high, she used this as a preparation for participating in the community, helping them build their confidence to perhaps take an outside class.

> I've done classes outside and it's way easier than this. I explained to them that if you go to a drop-in class at the Y, it's going to be easy for you now.

> For me, taking them out into the world…a lot of them are terrified to go to a [community] place and that's why we're going to the fitness center next Friday. They get a chance to get on the treadmill or elliptical so that if they join a club, they can have the confidence. It's one thing to tell them that we have a fitness center but to actually show them…

Interconnectedness: Kindness and Connecting Beyond the Self

> So the interconnectedness I talk about a lot, getting outside, connecting with other people, putting down your phone. That human or animal—that live connection is very important. Even when we are in the studio, I say, "breathe, then make your breath feel a part of the positive energy in the room." We are all connected to this peaceful environment or space. Letting them know and feel they are a part of this peaceful environment, that they are not just visitors or spectators—they are helping to create the environment, they are part of it. They can benefit from this kind of tweaking their perspective and being at peace.

This "web of interconnectedness" (Kabat-Zinn, 1990, p. 157) beyond the self is significant to the health of the individual and to the health of the planet. Kim helps students perceive and experience how they are all connected to each other, to the community, to the Earth. Her empathy and way of teaching in itself demonstrates kind, compassionate living—providing daily opportunities for students to witness how the smallest of things are sometimes connected to the most significant events (Kornfield, 2000). Kim's awareness of interconnectedness, of connecting beyond the self, past the classroom, and into the community also helps guide her in choosing the activities she offers to and participates in with the students.

> While we are whole ourselves as individual beings, we are also part of a larger whole, interconnected through our family and our friends and acquaintances to the larger society and ultimately to the whole of humanity and life on the planet. (Kabat-Zinn, 1990, p. 157)

On a regular basis, students are encouraged to share their day-to-day stories of when they have been kind to others in their family, the school, the community, or beyond. These stories are discussed and Kim probes students about what impact they think their actions or words might have and how it made them feel. Some of the activities students described included fundraising events for charity organizations, helping a neighbor shovel snow, and lending clothing to a friend to go to yoga class. Kim recalls when she taught students about Yoga Nidra[1] and shared her guided recording with them.

> Some girls have emailed me and I sent it [recording] to them and they are starting to use it at home. One student passed it on to her mom who suffers from anxiety and that just warms my heart and that's what it's all about.

Other activities that Kim promotes in class are "bring your own water bottle" and the "no-litter lunch." While sometimes throughout the semester Kim has to gently remind students not to bring plastic water bottles to class, she explains that she understands it is sometimes difficult to change a habit and they discuss the impact of water bottles on the planet. The difficulty they discuss is that when they forget their water bottle, they also remember how important it is to drink water for their own health, thus they buy water from the vending machine. This type of open, nonjudgmental discussion is important as it illustrates further issues that may have not been evident on the surface. It encourages students to look at the issue of drinking water from multiple perspectives, allows them to further question the "real" issue and understand that their input is valued. As a former high school teacher, it demonstrated for me how quickly I have previously rushed to judgment and thought of the students as just disrespectful, uncaring, or forgetful teenagers. As Kim reminded me, they hear more of what we say than we think.

In wisdom traditions, reciprocity reflects the belief that humans live interdependently with all forms of life, and our spiritual, emotional, social, and mental health is dependent upon our harmonious relationship with others and nature

(Hart, 1999). In Kim's class, these reciprocal relationships were demonstrated by the dynamic circle of teaching and learning, and giving and receiving (Tibbetts, Faircloth, Nee-Benham, & Pfeiffer, 2000). For example, some of Kim's previous students who are now in college were significantly impacted by what they learned in her H2O class and decided to "give back" to her current class.

> Having Alison come back I think is just awesome because she's a great example of starting out as a belly dancer in grade 10 (and hating it) and then finding tribal fusion. Now coming back to volunteer.... This girl wanting to come back and teach, inspiring people...if you can inspire people to pursue that...that's a happy thing. Or I had a student last year ask me where I got certified and she went last summer to get her yoga certification so that she could teach.

Students also participate in a Grade One Buddies program where they are partnered with a grade-one student from a neighboring elementary school. The interaction between these grade-10, -11, and -12 students and the grade ones is magical, and it brings out a level of compassion and patience by teenagers that Kim is always astonished to witness. What is even more enlightening for these high school students is the impact they have on their young buddies. The grade-one students are always so happy when they come; and when one of the high school students is absent from class, the other students present see the disappointment in their grade-one partner.

Part of the formal requirements for the course is completing a community volunteer activity sometime during the semester and sharing this experience with the class. Kim explains why this is an important part of the course:

> Citizenship, giving back, their volunteer hours...it's about being kind, being mindful, because we are all connected.

One of the most significant aspects of the concept of interconnectedness is that it is cultivated through mindfulness. Kim's empathetic and kind way of being with her students allows her to pay attention to what is right in front of her, to the vulnerable, impressionable young individuals in her classes. She believes this is key to the success of teaching in a holistic way:

> After having my car accident and everything...I called it the invisible pain.... Now I am very sympathetic to those students who come in and I wonder what invisible pain they have. It could be that they got laughed at when they were in junior high when they tried to dance. It could be an eating disorder. It could be depression. You don't know what they are dealing with, so you just want to have that empathy for them and realize that one of these activities could really help them.

> It's just having that understanding—you just have to be empathetic…. Have a sense of humor and you have to make working out fun. Phys. Ed was never fun for me—I had the power trip teacher. We need enthusiastic instructors who truly do see the benefit of this alternative approach. It's not about what you teach. It's about if you're going to go out and play Frisbee, how are you going to organize and do that with your students?

This kind, compassionate way of being requires a paradigm shift from the Cartesian dualism that is dominant in Western society where body and mind are separate, to the perspective that is common among wisdom traditions where body–mind–spirit are connected into a whole (Mehl-Madrona, 2005). It means that to maintain balance and harmony, we need to recognize the relationships that we form within ourselves and with others, understanding that we should approach the physical, mental, spiritual, and emotional in the same way. "We evolve through relationships" (Mehl-Madrona, 2005, p. 4); and we must remember that if we focus our relationships with our students to develop the physical over the other dimensions, we promote disharmony *within* our students, which leads to a state of unhealthy being and can lead to illness. Then what often happens in Western culture, because we consider mind and body separate, is that we turn to drugs to treat what is considered strictly a biological, physical problem (Robinson, 2008). Kind, compassionate living involves us building relationships with our students and recognizing the wholeness of their being.

> It's the human element—that's the difference, that's big…and then that empathy and that kids all come in with their issues. How can Phys. Ed be used as a tool to prevent some of their ailments instead of pills? Be proactive instead of reactive.

Building Community

Over time, Kim has realized that an important part of the notion of interconnectedness begins with purposeful actions within the classroom to help students experience a sense of community.

> When I started the circuit, I said, please don't think this is a bad thing. We are all in this together, we are all going to work hard, and this is going to make us feel better. As you go through it just breathe and feed off the energy in the room. I'm always talking about energy in the room.

It is especially important to help students try to connect with each other in a safe environment that resembles a small microcosm of society because, as Kim explains,

"Twenty-first-century learners"—that's the district's buzzword. But these 21st-century learners are not social and they're not connected. They are connected to their phones and their devices but unconnected to each other. So you can stay at home and do Wii dance in your bedroom by yourself or you can get out. So I say to them, you have to find that motivation and those friends to get you off the couch. That human connection, the physical sweating, the laughing, learning and having fun doing it—that's what's important.

Communicating and Sharing Stories

Pema Chodron (1994) believes that compassionate action requires us to "communicate from the heart" and that "all activities should be done with the intention of communicating" (p. 115). This intention involves "exchang[ing] oneself for other...it is to hear what's being said, to see the person who is in front of you" (p. 116). Kim believes that you must be willing to acknowledge the differences that exist between individuals (including the different perspectives among teachers and students), play together without needing to win, be open to other perspectives, and "that we are all in this together." Chodron (1994) says, "the process is the main thing, not the fruition" (p. 118) and "everybody needs someone to be there for them" (p. 119). Kim understands that many teachers do not like to show their vulnerabilities and avoid becoming "too caring" or "involved" because they feel the need to fix or solve a problem. However, as Chodron (1994) points out, "sometimes there's nothing to be said and nothing to be done...the deepest communication of all is just to be there" (p. 120). Kim always tries to remember to see, feel, and listen to herself and recognize her own pain and suffering, realize that the others around her may share the same pain although the source of pain may be different. She shares her thoughts and experiences with students—whether it is about success or failure, pain or joy, acceptance or rejection—showing a level of "humanness" that contributes to the inclusive, positive environment that exists in this class. It fosters positive relationships and encourages students to live kind, compassionate lives.

Kim often shares and communicates personal stories about people, experiences, and events to provide metaphors for understanding and to help students to connect on an emotional and spiritual level; otherwise, she says, "they just go through the motions" and "shut off." Kuyvenhoven (2005) believes "storytelling is a learning event and communicates a body of knowledge dependent on presence" (p. 135). You need to relate what they are doing in class to everyday life, and storytelling often sparks a connection to something within an individual, commonalities of how we feel or experiences beyond the walls of the classroom.

> I share my stories…I talk about my body, my history, my stress, how I've adapted my life. I let students know that they may feel like they're going to crash and burn and life can be a marathon. I tell them about how I went so hard into coaching and so hard into all this stuff that I just collapsed. So pacing yourself…finding different activities that you can do for life without killing yourself. So we need to also find the mental, spiritual exercises, to go with the physical exercises for students to partake in.

Mehl-Madrona (2005) reminds us that the

> telling and retelling of stories is the powerful means by which cultures of families and communities are formed and maintained, national identities are preserved, problem-solving skills are taught, and moral values are instilled. Stories can inspire, uplift, and transform their listeners, or they can belittle, humiliate, and drive their listeners to despair. Stories get our attention to teach us things we will never forget. (pp. 1–2)

As Kim describes it:

> I tell them stories…I have had activities that came very easily too, but there were also a lot of things that didn't come easily to me. I just remember being terrified of taking figure skating at the Glenora Club and being the largest kid in gymnastics class—never being enrolled in dance because I was too big for it. So they just put me in basketball. I was always the biggest and I was usually that kid that didn't fit in. So I just have this empathy. So when we are starting a new activity, even when it was traditional Phys. Ed, I would ask, "How many of you hate skating?" So then, are you able to laugh at yourself like I did? And then they're usually fine with it, and so just putting it out there—I'm not going to be the best gymnast in the room but just give it a try and get through it. I just know what it's like to not be good at something. When I started belly dancing—how foolish I felt and just having my male instructor coming up and being supportive and saying good for you! Even if you don't want to share a personal story, just identifying the fact that not everybody's going to be good at this activity…this is a lifelong activity and we're all here trying some things, so give it your best shot.

Archibald (2008) explains, "stories have the power to make our hearts, minds, bodies and spirits work together" (p. 21). Kim knows her stories—both actions and words—may not be understood by her students right now. It may be several months or years before they take any meaning for themselves, but she feels it is still important to tell the story because in time, perhaps they will remember the story and it will be helpful for them.

Balance

Wholeness is "about the incorporation of all aspects of life and the giving of attention and energy to each aspect within ourselves and the universe around us" (Hart, 2008, p. 134). When we promote and support students to be healthy and well, we focus on a balance of the physical, emotional, social, and spiritual dimensions of the individual. Too often with a sport-technique model of physical education (Kirk, 2010), there is a focus on one aspect (physical) to the detriment of the other parts (Hart, 2008).

Connected to the notion of maintaining balance of the whole self, body–mind–spirit, is how to set up a program that aligns with this philosophy. Kim explains that what guides her planning is balance—a balance of realistic, affordable activities that then can promote a wholeness of living. In most physical education curricula across Canada, program documents encourage teachers to choose a *variety* of physical activities. It is important to note, that *balance* is not the same as *variety*. You can have a program with a variety of activities (e.g., games, individual/dual activities, alternate environment, dance, gymnastics) that still does not promote balance. Having a balanced program means that whatever activities you choose, how we present these activities, and how we participate in these activities should go beyond just the physical, and encourage balance within (emotional, physical, mental, and spiritual) and harmony among all living things (Hart, 2008).

> So what guides my planning is showing the students affordable, practical, fun, and accessible activities and practices. What we try to do every week is balance and different things—cardio/strength, creative dance, yoga, games, theory, our grade-one buddies, or line dancing or something like that. So every week I just want to have a balance of things that goes beyond just physicality but helps them, you know, emotionally, spiritually.

> So a lot of this program too, I think, is introducing any skill level, any body type, any person to these activities…we want our [program] to be open, we don't want it to be elitist or turned into a fashion show, we don't want it to be a Lulu catwalk. We want every student—male or female, no matter what his or her experience—to feel comfortable taking this course.

While part of that balance involves choosing activities that promote a wholeness of living, Kim also believes it is important to connect into the community to have key role models and instructors speak to and lead students through various holistic activities. Whom you choose as a guest and to interact and dialogue with students should be done with care and attentiveness to the philosophy of the course and needs of students. Kim not only tries to ensure that the guest's message is positive, holistic, and empowering, she also wants the activity to be something that students can then relate to or incorporate in their teenage worlds and beyond.

> So I love having Georgette Reed come in and share her story about being overweight and being lost and about not fitting in, because I think in some point of our lives we've all felt like that. So bringing in strong leaders, and especially women, in this course and the fact that she can bench press more than any man. So her redefinition of what a woman is, I love that for the students. And the highlight from that is the feedback that I got from the class the next day was amazing. They cried, they laughed, they were inspired—they just loved her energy…the gleam in her eyes, her magic when she talks—they really liked that.

To Test or Not to Test: Merging Poles

Throughout the semester, Kim and I struggled with the physical education department's requirement of fitness testing for students. The base fitness-testing day took place in September and the follow-up in December. Since a key philosophical principle of the course is about not judging each other, not measuring people against standards to determine worth, the one-time fitness testing idea with results submitted to the department database was problematic. Achieving wellness cannot take place on one day at one time with one test. It should be an ongoing process where students become aware of how their bodies feel when they are healthy and well.

The fitness testing issue challenged us on many fronts and precipitated discussion about the value of this traditional approach, what students actually learn about being healthy and connecting with their bodies with this method, and what type of "testing" (if any) aligned more appropriately to a holistic approach. Kim commented that in the past when she did not include fitness testing in the course, students did not necessarily have awareness about their level of fitness. So perhaps one value is to raise awareness about this one component of their overall wellness.

> So I have to do this testing and I'm still wondering if it's beneficial. But I do see the relevance.

> What I do see, because I was dead set against it, but because some of them botched out at level 2—that's a startling lack of fitness. So I do see the point in this for the fitness stuff.

Empirically, fitness testing measures *physical* fitness and usually includes both health (cardiovascular, muscular strength and endurance, flexibility) and skill-related (agility, balance, coordination, reaction time, power, and speed) abilities. Safrit (1990) notes "although components of physical fitness can be identified and tested...a unified indicator of one's true fitness status can only be approximated. It cannot be determined precisely" (p. 10). Thus the question is: what does fitness testing tell us about how to be healthy, how to be well? Is it a necessary component in a wellness-oriented physical education curriculum? For school-aged children and youth, research suggests that fitness testing in physical education settings is questionable in promoting healthy active lifestyles. As Cale and Harris (2009) explain,

> much of the fitness testing carried out in PE may well represent a misdirected effort in the promotion of healthy lifestyles and physical activity, and that PE time could therefore be better spent. There appears to be little evidence that fitness tests promote healthy lifestyles and physical activity, motivate young people, and develop the knowledge, understanding and skills that are important to engagement in an active lifestyle. To the contrary, there is evidence to suggest that fitness testing may be counterproductive to the goal of promoting physical activity for some youngsters. (p. 105)

In Kim's situation, she was required to complete the fitness testing protocol. She understood that it was not a measurement of a student's overall wellness, and it could potentially have a negative impact on students' emotional, spiritual, and mental wellbeing, as well as their overall motivation to participate in future activities. Consequently what became the focus surrounding fitness testing in her class was not the scores, but the process—preparing for the day, completing the challenge, how to interpret the results, and how it feels during and after participating.

> I hate throwing kids into fitness testing, so my approach and whole philosophy is don't compare yourself with anyone else. I use myself as an example...I can't touch my toes, I can't do different things and that's okay, that's my body. Certain people can dance, some can't. But that's the thing, and I'm trying to push that so that when we do the fitness test and that kind of thing, they're not feeling bad about themselves. Do what you can and we would like everyone to improve by the end of the year.

But then I am like, this is a mental test too…this isn't the Olympics, don't stress. We even did the exercises in a circuit before so that wasn't the first time they were doing the side lunges or the flexibility. I would never just walk in and play the tape and throw students into it because it is so intimidating.

When I first started this course, I didn't do a cardio component with the students and I realized that when we would go out there they were still out of shape. So now I prepped them for a month before we did it and I try to explain to them why we're doing it.

The beep test…those people that go out at 1 or 2 are the people that I'm really concerned with. In ten years they may not be able to climb a set of stairs without being out of breath. So whether they get up to 6,7,8,9….That's going to depend on body type and genetics and their activity level but I know [student] will likely drop out at 1.6 again because she doesn't care. So it is testing so many other things and that's why I say it is a mental test too.

At the end of the semester, Kim was still uneasy about the role of fitness testing in this class. She recognized that it could be useful for helping students get an idea of their level of fitness, but questioned if it is the right fitness testing for this course. Furthermore, it highlights only one component of one dimension of wellness (the physical), de-emphasizing the importance of the other dimensions of the whole self.

Michelle:	So what other things can you do to monitor physical fitness?
Kim:	I would like to see a class set of heart rate monitors so doing that at the beginning of the year with some of the workouts and recording throughout, and then at the end of the year, recovery time and so on. That would be ideal.
Michelle:	That's about process? It's ongoing monitoring and it helps them understand and see the heart rate that is going down with the same volume of work, then you are seeing an improvement in fitness.
Kim:	Then it is done more consistently throughout the semester. Like the one girl who had the asthma attack on the second test and one girl didn't have breakfast, so it's not accurate.
Michelle:	It's ongoing.
Kim:	And it's a life skill…taking that information when they don't have a heart rate monitor and being able to feel it themselves. They don't need a heart rate monitor on because they will know where their optimum level is based on their breathing, and eventually they will be able to feel that. So that's eventually where I would like to see it going.

(Non)Assessment of Wellness

It's this constant connection back to their bodies…no matter what the activities, whether it's yoga, dance, circuits, games, even when you debrief [from guest speakers]—it's connecting into their emotions and their spiritual health…and when we go see the grade ones, how does that make you feel when you go see them?

How do you assess this?

All this stuff, they are adjusting their diet, getting rid of caffeine, relaxing before bed, and that's success. But again, how do I measure that…. Doing Yoga Nidra at home? Do I give them a mark for that?

How do you assess this? Do you need to?

For today's student…it's "how do I get a better mark?" It's not learning. We talked about [a colleague] and her assessment and kids focusing on marks not the process. How do I get a 90, not how do I become a good writer, a healthy person? You don't want kids in this class…how do I get 100—if I do a perfect downward dog, do I get 100? No, it's process, practicing—not the results.

How do you measure wellness?

What about guiding their own practice in yoga? We talked about the physical checklist of what you need to do to do for the physical posture but then there's the mental, spiritual, emotional, mind–body–spirit connection. So assessment?… big question mark!

How do you measure wellness? What do you measure?

It's hard to measure the impact on students today. The effects and appreciation won't be realized until their 20s and 30s. I know down the road…they will tap into this stuff.

How do you measure wellness? When do you assess it? Who evaluates your wellness? Who decides?

The topic of assessment was a major dilemma that surfaced throughout the semester. Kim has spent the last five years wrestling with this dilemma about assessing and evaluating students' in a holistic health class. What message does it leave with the student about taking care of their whole self if you are judging them with external standards at one particular time? If they have improved their spiritual health exponentially during the semester, you may only begin to see the impact of that on their overall wellness as they move toward being a more balanced, healthy individual. After considerable discussion, we decided to keep the question open and share what we have learned so far. Overall, what we do know is that again, assessment also needs to be mindful. Students need to learn how to notice, to pay attention to their bodies, to be able to connect body–mind–spirit. This comes full circle to the curriculum, the journey, the process.

Beyond Physicality

Assessment strategies that focus on physical performance and impose external interpretations of the affective domain exclude the wholeness of the individual. Assessment should be a dialogical and dialectical process between the teacher and student that includes the mental, physical, emotional, and spiritual dimensions of the whole person.

> I'm going to ask them how they feel they did and to give themselves a mark on yoga—how well they were able to concentrate and focus during the Savasana and did they actually relax or did they just fall asleep or were they fidgety? And maybe with the other exercises…did you feel like you got physically fitter, emotionally better, spiritually more aware, and just how has it changed you, your outlook?

Individual

Students need to be aware of their own wellness and learn how to assess what that means for themselves as individuals.

> I think the common theme even with the fitness testing the other day is about just bettering yourself and not competing with others. That's basically the whole premise—don't look around and compete. It's about shaking your hips when you're belly dancing and feeling liberated…we're all in it together…we're all just participating, no one looking around at each other.

Ongoing Mindful Practice and Reflection

Assessment and evaluation practices not only need to be ongoing throughout the semester but need to foster the ability of students to develop discipline for ongoing practice and be able to self-assess their day-to-day wellbeing. This is part of mindful practice.

> There is no end point to any of this; it's a practice, your yoga, your eating habits, everything. And we're all going to have off days and we talk about that all the time. At the end of class—how many of you could focus today, how many of you couldn't? And it's different every day…. So I think it's more a reflection, like a "stop and evaluate."

> The healthy habits logbooks…the girls found it useful. Again that is mindful…. I like the fact that it's about the sleep patterns, it's water, and eating habits. And there are so many light bulb [moments]—when they realize, oh my God, I didn't drink water for three days, my sleep or this or that—it lets me know too because I understand why this girl never has any energy. She can't do the circuit because she didn't have breakfast or lunch.

> The laughing and the smiling and it [line dance] was so much fun, and then I had them feel their heart rate. We didn't time it or anything but I said feel that! You're laughing and you're getting a workout in. We even had to open the windows and turn the fan on.

Holistic Health Option (H2O): The New Health and Physical Education (HPE) Program?

On occasion we put this course in the context of what it was not. Emphatically, Kim believes that H2O is not a traditional physical education course. Teaching a wellness curriculum ironically highlights what is wrong with most of today's physical education classes. By focusing so much on sport, technique, efficiencies, execution, and physical fitness, we actually encourage unhealthy, inactive lifestyles instead of the "healthy active lifestyles" (Alberta Education, 2000) that curricular documents state as the goal of physical education (Kilborn, Lorusso, & Francis, 2015). She recognizes that physical education courses (including Sports Performance in Alberta) have many pieces—activities, sports, skills, fitness principles, nutrition, leadership, cooperation, "do it daily"—but lack a wholeness perspective.

> It's the human element, that's the difference, that's big…teaching this way has to be humanizing—these are human beings in front of us, it's not about how many balls they can get in the target.

As the province of Alberta where Kim teaches is in the process of redesigning their senior high physical education and health curricula, Kim believes that if the intention is to promote wellness for our students, this course could be a good example of how to set up a new Health and Physical Education program of studies for the province.

· 6 ·

PEDAGOGICAL MOMENTS
SYNTHESIZED

Learn from the vastness of the open space
The tickle of the wind on the leaves
The effortless flight of the winged
The awe of the sacred mountains with all their might
Place our bodies, minds and spirits within the wisdom of the Earth.
— MICHELLE KILBORN, (N.D.), INSPIRED FROM HARTKE,
1990, PP. XVI–XVIII

A curriculum of wellness is based in understanding, moving beyond a text-based view to a *currere*-based perspective that is active, dynamic, and contextual. Irwin (2006) reminds us,

> excursion means *excurrere*, meaning to run outward, while *recurrere* means running back to the course (both in Latin). Excursions become those trips seeking understanding beyond the original course of action, while recursions circle back before venturing outward again. Implicit within the root word *currere* is the notion of running forward. Thus curriculum is and needs to be a course of action that advances understanding. (p. 77)

Part of circling back home on our journey then means (re)turning to the field of physical education to add a new conversation to the existing dialogue among teachers and scholars. But how do we explain our "results"? What is the answer to our main question about teaching a curriculum of wellness? Kim reminded me there is no "answer," there is no one solution. It truly is about the journey, and instead of looking for the answer, or an end product, focus on the journey—the "how" not the "what." Interpreting the pedagogical moments along the way allows you to see that the journey of life (curriculum) itself, being a teacher itself, is pedagogical. This requires you to look at who you are, the way you are, and why you do what you do the way you do. Focusing on who you are as a teacher and the way you teach allows you to question your own assumptions and be open to multiple perspectives. Thus, it starts with the self. Ending our preoccupations with our quest for the best performance, the one right way, the answer to solve an issue, allows an opportunity for a deeper understanding of the real dilemmas we face. If we are truly concerned about the health and wellness of our children and youth, it is time to peel away the layers of our individual and collective identities, and recover the unity of body–mind–spirit. We must face what is presently in front us—a mechanistic, disconnected, dualistic view of the body—and begin again so that we may understand our students as whole beings.

We understand meaning making is situated and is dependent upon each individual's own interaction with the stories we have told. Our desire to end our (con)textual representation of a curriculum of wellness in physical education at this point was very strong. However, inquiry, teaching, and learning exists in the space between the two poles, and wellbeing depends on dynamic movement, unity, balance, and harmony. As such, we must trust that presenting a more positivistic summary (complete with four fragmented "themes") of what it means to teach in this way will flow together with the experience of the ontological, axiological, cosmological, and epistemological knowledge(s) that were expressed in our previous stories.

There are four "big ideas" that I am offering as discussion points for people to go out on their own excursions, their own journeys, and return home. Based on Kim's experiences with H2O and this inquiry, to teach in this way it is important that you first start with the self, reconceptualize the notion of curriculum, view teaching as a way of being (not the act of teaching), and understand children as whole beings. Again, it is difficult to compartmentalize these ideas as each one of them flows among, in between, and within the other. As such, readers may find that some ideas grouped under one heading may actually belong in all headings or perhaps seem to belong in another. The point here is not to wrap everything up in a nice, neat package, but to invoke a sense of wonder, a pondering that will allow us to perhaps challenge our own assumptions, be *un*comfortable with the status quo, and dare to see things otherwise. So for those of you, like myself, who love to organize, arrange, itemize, and so on, try to breathe and accept this place and space in between and sit with it.

It Starts with the Self

Rose Auger, a Cree medicine woman from the Driftpile Reserve in Alberta, shares:

> Human development is the finding of your identity by looking at your history, your roots. It's a way of life that guides you and helps you to know the right thing to do.... We have to relate to what's around us—be it a tree, a blade of grass, or clear spring water.... People's beliefs are layered around them, and the layers are hard to peel off because they are so tough from years of reinforcement. Just like an onion, the layers must be gently peeled away until the soft heart at the centre is exposed. (Meili, 1991, p. 23)

Within five years of teaching, the technical, "pressure-to-win" way of teaching/coaching was instrumental in Kim's state of being unwell—mentally, physically, emotionally, and spiritually. She designed and began teaching H2O but still continued to coach, and consequently just *delivered* the course to students. It was not until she was forced to take the time to look within and examine her own life that her perspectives about teaching began to shift. When she began taking yoga and belly-dance classes, and learning about alternative philosophies for health, physical education, and wellness, she began to see the potential in sharing this with her students. Teaching was no longer solely about meeting the learning outcomes; it became about meeting her students, sharing stories with her students, dancing with her students, laughing with her students, and living the curriculum *together with* her students. She understood that her own way of living and taking care of herself was the most important factor to being able to help others live healthfully. Her way of being a teacher is her way of being in life.

I am not suggesting that all teachers of physical education do not choose healthy habits for themselves—many are conscientious about fitness and nutrition, and very focused on maintaining the physical body. What I am suggesting is instead of looking *at* the self, look *in* the self and recognize the whole person—body, mind, and spirit. I have no doubt that we are genuinely concerned about the health of our children and youth; however, I believe we continue to look objectively to address the issue. The Dalai Lama (2001) asks us to consider this:

> Violence...growing numbers of young people addicted to drugs and alcohol, sui-
> cide...unlike sufferings of old age, sickness and death, none of these problems is by
> nature inevitable. Nor are they due to any lack of knowledge. When we think care-
> fully, we see that they are all ethical problems.... We can point to something more
> fundamental: a neglect of what I call our inner dimension. (p. 15)

The Dalai Lama (2001) is calling for a spiritual reawakening, and we in the physical education world may want to consider this and start with ourselves, understanding that we are dialectically linked to our students and the greater community. Irwin (2006) explains how the pedagogy of the self is often ne-glected and specifically addresses how "educators usually focus their care on others; yet if they wish to truly care for others, it is vitally important for them to care for themselves first" (p. 75). Kumar (2013) believes "it is the self and its interactions that form society, and unless the fundamental unit—self—transforms there is no possibility of a profound social change" (p. 114). In a session at the 2011 Canadian Society for the Study of Education conference, Dwayne Donald, a Canadian scholar on Indigenous perspectives in curricu-lum and education, reminded us that to participate in a community (locally, nationally, and globally) and understand what is needed to make change, we must first attend to our own stories.

This first-person ontology is very much needed in physical education research. Kirk (2013) states, "physical educators lack a perspective on their field" (p. 220). I would suggest that for physical education to consider any type of reform, we must have perspective *in* ourselves and our field, not *on* them. This will require greater acceptance of research that considers individ-ual and personal subjectivities in order to extend our understanding of the collective. As Kumar (2013) explains, understanding and transforming our consciousness is critical, but it is important that we consider both individ-ual and collective consciousness together—"superficially, certainly individ-ual consciousness and collective consciousness seem distinct, but deeply, our consciousness, like our universe, does not have any divisions" (p. 116). This means it would be wise to not separate narrative, autobiographical, storytell-ing, and life history inquiry from the collective situation. This is not to un-dermine the work that some physical education scholars are doing in this area (i.e., Armour, 2006; Evans, 2004; Ovens & Fletcher, 2014; Maivorsdotter & Lundvall, 2009; Schaefer, 2013; S. Smith, 1992; Sparkes, 1994, 1995, 1999, 2002; Sparks & Templin, 1992). My point is that the ontological knowledge of physical education teachers needs to be valued and more should be encour-aged to share their stories and perspectives of their own experiences.

Reconceptualizing Curriculum in Physical Education

To understand a reconceptualist notion of curriculum as *currere*, Pinar "called on those involved in educational work (professors, administrators, teachers, and students) to engage in theorizing. Individuals engaged in theorizing strive to understand the present by excavating their pasts and imagining possible futures" (Schubert, 2009, p. 137). Reconceptualized theorizing helps broaden the discussion from curriculum development (and implementation) to curriculum studies that "embrace[s] multiple texts or discourse communities (historical, political or ideological, racial, gendered aesthetic, biographical, autobiographical, phenomenological, poststructural and postmodern, theological, and international" (Schubert, 2009, p. 138). This type of theorizing has seldom been recognized by traditional and conceptual empiricist curriculum developers (which are the dominant perspectives in physical education), as it does not support the normally expected generalized curriculum packages, programs, models, kits, and designs sold en masse to educational institutions. Instead, this type of theorizing involves teacher educators taking the living process of sharing perspectives and possibilities (not a static product) back to teacher education programs and encouraging teachers to engage in theorizing with their own students where questions are asked, the world is pondered, and hopes of a better universe are realized (Schubert, 2009, p. 138).

While physical education scholars Jewett, Bain, and Ennis (1995) characterize curriculum as *praxis*, where theory and practice are interactive and not separate, their work is still largely positioned within a traditional curriculum perspective where theorizing is for purposes of developing conceptual frameworks and models that can then be applied to or administered to students. And while their exploration of value orientations in curriculum (disciplinary mastery, social reconstruction, learning process, self-actualization, and ecological validity) present different perspectives and provide an opening for discussion about how we interact with curriculum, these are still presented in a fragmented, compartmentalized way. They encourage those working in the physical education field to recognize the importance of making values explicit in curriculum work (Jewett & Bain, 1985, p. 25), but infer a nondialectic, either-or approach that is somewhat reductionistic, "convert[ing] *a* way of life into *the* way of life" (Aoki, as cited in Pinar & Irwin, 2005, p. 347). A reconceptualized understanding of curriculum is simultaneous in nature, where we see, experience, and co-construct meaning with the power of double or multiple vision (Aoki, as cited in Pinar & Irwin, 2005).

Once Kim embraced the truth that living well involves knowing yourself in a holistic manner, she found that her ability as a teacher to make curriculum come alive was significantly enhanced. Her focus is on taking care of herself and others. Others in this case are her students and her students' others, understanding that we are all connected. This collaborative inquiry and the insights we gained provided an aperture into the world of teaching a curriculum of wellness in physical education. Teaching in this way is possible because curriculum was reconceptualized and considered a journey where the focus was on "how" not "what," and an acceptance that it is an ongoing, dialectical, dialogical journey *with* the students.

Kim's wellness way of being a teacher is difficult to realize if curriculum is considered to be the checklist or manual for the knowledge/skill factory in a neo-liberalist education system, where students are mass produced to meet certain standards in a specified time period (inspired by Ken Robinson's "Changing Paradigms" lecture, 2008). Nurturing a wholeness of being is ongoing *practice*, it is open ended and students will learn in their own time. We understand this notion through Kim's experiences with past students and herself, in that some of what we are "learning" in H2O in high school does not manifest itself into action until much later. Smith (2011a) reminds us,

> As part of wisdom understanding, the kairotic sense of time is of enormous relevance in teaching, but again, unrecognized in almost all educational theory today. It involves a recognition that things have their time in a way that cannot be delivered chronometrically. Some students simply take longer to appreciate some things than others. (pp. 176–177)

This openness and responsiveness involves teachers helping students to be "self-reflective in their thinking, assumptions, and values" (Kumar, 2013, p. 99) and "sets learners free to explore, seek, search, discover, invent, and experiment" (p. 100).

A curriculum of wellness is also interconnected and understands the "journey of life" (Grumet, 1980) to be circular. It respects that who we are and how we are as individuals is intricately linked to all other living things, and to the Earth. This reciprocity is not limited to what is happening in the "classroom," and demands that we connect into a broader understanding of what and where pedagogical opportunities exist in curriculum. Maxine Greene believes this calls for an individual to be present and aware of oneself, of one's whole experience—"it calls for an awareness of the process of living in which we are all involved, which emphasizes our interconnectedness" (Pautz, 1998, p. 30). It is of moral nature and "involves taking responsibility for one's life within the wider, interconnected set of communities in which one lives" (p. 31). When you live a curriculum of wellness with your students, you are actively aware of issues, problems, and dilemmas that arise in the lives of your students and yourself and face them with "depth, with creativity and originality" (Pautz, 1998, p. 31). Understanding these dialectical, dialogical, and reciprocal relationships with ourselves, students, and all living things forms an environment where teaching and learning is inside students' everyday experiences, not outside.

A curriculum of wellness guided by wisdom encourages wholeness that can refer to many aspects of curriculum, such as valuing all ways of knowing (epistemology, axiology, ontology, cosmology), nondualism, dimensions of the self (mental, emotional, physical, spiritual), and self and other. The idea of a more (w)holistic approach to physical education curriculum has gained some attention over the years but still remains a fringe discussion waiting to be realized within the school community. To further explain, I will first begin with physical education's current curriculum situation and then address how a reconceptualized curriculum of wellness must honor wholeness, within physical education, across all curricula, and in connection with the community.

The dominant goal within most physical education curriculum around the world is clearly identified as acquiring the knowledge, skills, and attitudes for healthy active living (or lifestyle, or for life) (Hardman, 2008, 2013; Kilborn, 2011; Kilborn, Lorusso & Francis, 2015). What does this really mean and do we really mean it? Health (1550, O.E. *hælþ*) means "wholeness, a being whole, sound or well" (health, n.d.). Life (O.E. dative *lif*) means "existence, lifetime, way of life, condition of being a living thing" (life, n.d.). It is clear that our intended goal for physical education is to help children and youth live a way of life to be whole, to be well. However, there seems to be a disconnect between this planned curriculum and the living curriculum. Hardman and Marshall (2005) confirm,

> A major issue is that of the relevance and quality of physical education curricula around the globe. In some parts of the world physical education curricula are undergoing change with signs that its purpose and function are being redefined to accommodate broader life-long educational outcomes. Nevertheless, there remains an orientation towards sports-dominated competitive performance-related activity programmes. (p. 7)

So why is it such a challenge for physical education to change this competitive sports-dominated approach? Smith (2008c) addresses how the impact of market logic based on competition sets up a system of "haves" and "have-nots" where "comparative advantage" and the "victimization of the weak" (p. 42) perpetuates a commodified, disconnected world void of compassion and empathy. This issue has great significance to the health and wellness of children and youth, as it sets up an environment of despair where students without "abilities" live in a lonely world of rejection, low self-esteem and frustration. The symptoms of this neoliberal and neoconservative agenda are displayed in the increasing incidents of mental health issues, violence, and substance abuse among youth, and physical inactivity (Tremblay et al., 2010).

This social Darwinism world of competition to obtain status and power is at the root of sport and a major influence on school physical education programs. Bourdieu's (1998) description of gaining short-term profits at any cost, the individualism of performance, and a competition-based reward system are most noteworthy in the context of physical education. In fact, these concepts highlight some of the reasons why physical education curriculum reform efforts may have fallen short. While a more holistic approach to physical education would likely result in better long-term health outcomes for students, there is more short-term capital in using physical education classes to identify individual athletes who will then contribute to a winning franchise (not team)—ultimately leading to increased status, recognition, and profit. Unfortunately this sets up an educational environment that rewards individual performance and actually leads to an overall decrease in participation, as those who do not have physical capital are marginalized. The vision of material wealth associated with professional sport helps perpetuate the Cartesian dualism of body and mind being separate and ironically often leads to inactivity, injury, and subsequent health issues. These negative trends for young people are further fueled by the product-driven, extrinsically based education system that places more value on the accumulation of knowledge and commodities. Patel (2009) explains that while the basic human needs (housing, food, water) do have an impact on health, having more wealth does not increase happiness. So, as we push our students to know more so that they can acquire more, we are actually damaging their physical, emotional, and spiritual health. The long-term impact of this neoliberalist market-driven mentality is a population of students who are not active, have become disconnected from their bodies, and look outside themselves for happiness. All of this feeds the commercialization of health. These are powerful forces to work against when seeking a change in how we teach physical education.

When people, governments, and corporations pursue "as much of a given thing as they can get" (Patel, 2009, p. 27) in a market society, it affects the wellbeing of all living things. This undying loyalty to a market-driven world inherited from generations past values the objective and excludes the subjective. By ignoring the subjective, we fail to attend to other dimensions that foster better holistic health (e.g., social, emotional, spiritual health) (Lu, Tito, & Kentel, 2009). This subjective awareness, as discussed by some physical education scholars (Arnold, 1979; Bain, 1990; Halas 2011; Kalyn, 2006; Lloyd, 2011; Rintala, 1991; Salter 2000; Whitehead, 1990), is an important consideration for curriculum in physical education and an important concept common among wisdom traditions. Mindfulness and stillness are required to prevent spinning out of control (Welwood, 1992) and to connect—body, mind, spirit—to the earth. When we practice stillness, we are better able to pay attention to the present (composed of the regressive and progressive moments) and only then can we begin to (re)conceptualize curriculum in physical education and consider a wellness approach.

There are a number of education jurisdictions that have started moving in this direction and there are four specific examples I will highlight, as they demonstrate a regard for curriculum as a journey and some aspects of a curriculum of wellness (e.g., unity, balance, and wholeness). The first example is an overall whole-school approach called "health promoting schools"; the second involves a wellness approach in a New Mexico school; the third is Scotland's physical education curriculum; and finally Australia's work on a salutogenic approach.

While the health promoting schools approach is not specifically about physical education curriculum, it recognizes that learning happens beyond the specific subject area curricula and that students are whole beings in and out of school. It recognizes the interconnectedness of individuals and communities and seeks to restore balance within and among people. Health promoting schools seek to connect the whole child to the whole school, to the whole family, and to the whole community. Health promoting schools consider education and learning, healthy environments, school health services, partnerships with families and communities, and policies—which together form the "whole school approach enhancing both the health and educational outcomes of children and adolescents through learning and teaching experiences initiated in the schools" (International Union for Health Promotion and Education [IUHPE], 2010, p. 5). This approach respects the situatedness of the student and takes into consideration the social and cultural context of their lives. The real challenge with health promoting schools is that often the impetus for the approach being "implemented" is rooted in political and economic motivations from policymakers far removed from the school environment. The other challenge is bringing together the fragmented societal sectors, such as health, education, social services, and child and youth services, to be able to speak the same language and understand the life world of an individual student. While not perfect, the health promoting schools approach is a start. At the very least it provides an alternate vision for individuals to consider in their progressive moments while they analyze and synthesize the present back into the whole.

Silva, Arlyn, and Beenen (2008) discuss a philosophy of wellness that has been developed at the Native American Community Academy in New Mexico. This school's wellness philosophy incorporates a holistic approach that considers the social, emotional, physical, intellectual, and community relationship for each student. This wellness perspective uses the medicine wheel and emphasizes the importance of balance of the components of wellness and how these are always interconnected. The authors outline what this philosophy "looks like" and describe a typical day that involves a morning circle gathering, Personal Wellness classes that focus on the belief that "healthy bodies create a healthy community and environment," other wellness classes that teach youth how to reduce stress through active meditative practices, and science and language arts classes with garden projects that provide an opportunity to reconnect with traditional cultural practices.

Scotland's new "Curriculum for Excellence" education policy positions health and wellbeing as a high priority in the education system and recognizes physical education as "'an area of the curriculum which, exceptionally, needs greater priority to support the health and wellbeing of young people in Scotland' (Scottish Executive, 2004, p. 1)" (Thornburn, Jess, & Atencio, 2011, p. 386). The physical education curriculum itself focuses on learning experiences that are developmentally appropriate, inclusive, connect across the school curriculum, and are lifewide—"across all the different sectors of a child's life" (Thornburn, Jess, & Atencio, 2011, p. 387). This new curriculum will require teachers to consider mental, emotional, social, and physical wellbeing as part of their way of teaching and still meet specific standards for physical education, activity, and sport skills.

A salutogenic approach is considered strength based rather than the traditional deficit model used in the promotion and education of healthy active living. This approach in physical and health education curriculum "serves the role of fostering the competence of all students in order to construct a productive, harmonious, and healthy society within which individuals can enjoy quality of life (McCuaig & Hay, 2012, p. 287). McCuaig, Quennerstedt, and Macdonald (2013) further describe specific components of this type of curriculum, including a focus on the promotion of healthy living rather than disease prevention; a multidimensional view of healthy living that encompasses physical, social, mental, spiritual, environmental, and community dimensions; an understanding of health as dynamic—"always in the process of becoming" (p. 113); the view that health is something more than the absence of disease; acknowledgment of "humans as active agents, living in relation to their environment" (p. 113); and recognition of health as a "prerequisite for living a good life" (p. 113) not an end goal.

Thornburn, Jess, and Atencio (2011) acknowledge that the changes have provoked discussions about how to think differently about curriculum and "more precisely inquiring into what it means to be physically educated" (p. 396). However, it is important to build this from a collective narrative so that teachers subjectively accept new ideas about teaching rather than just becoming familiar with them.

While a different perspective for physical education curriculum is important, it is a moot concept if teachers treat it objectively outside themselves and fail to embody curriculum as an active, dynamic journey. Thus, how we view teaching is paramount to the task of realizing a curriculum of wellness.

Teaching as a Way of Being

Kim's inquiry process was concerned primarily with the questions: Who am I as a teacher? How does the way I am as a teacher affect how I teach? This perspective helps us distinguish "the act of teaching from *being* a teacher" (Feldman, 2009, p. 381). In educational philosophy, this idea of human *becoming* is more than just learning and experiencing the world; it includes understanding the "full situatedness of the individuals and their acknowledgements of their projects" (Feldman, 2009, p. 383).

It is important to realize though, that situatedness involves more than just the idea of context. Being situated takes into consideration the cultural environment and the influences of traditions, customs, institutions, and beliefs on what we do in a given situation. It also takes into account human interaction between the teacher and students, where the teacher is more than just the "knower," and the actions carried out are a result of the teacher's past, present, mood, and expectations combined with the culture, traditions, customs, and purposes of the situation. The characteristic of situatedness problematizes traditional modes of inquiry where teaching *practice* is emphasized rather than *being*. This practice focus infers that the teacher is separate from the situation in which she/he is teaching, which results in a disconnect that can be alienating and oppressive. As such wisdom-guided inquiry must reflect what happens when people explore their way of *being* a teacher.

This type of inquiry "recognizes that the subject of the research is one's own being" (Feldman, 2002, p. 242). This is important for physical educators as the nature of our discipline is focused on practice (related to *techne*) guided by preconceived activities and standards of performance. The idea of teaching as "a way of being" allows us to consider practice differently, as *phronesis*.

I reviewed Aristotle's three modes of knowledge in Chapter 1 to provide a greater understanding of the unique opportunity for a different way of thinking about "practice" in physical education. Upon analysis of the theoretical and nontheoretical forms of knowledge, it is evident how each plays a role in today's physical education classroom. Physical education's fundamental philosophy of body-as-machine lends itself to the productive disciplines where the *techne* disposition provides the ideal body image that is "so powerful that it dominates the action and directs it towards the given end" (Carr & Kemmis, 1986, pp. 32–33). This "means-end" perspective neglects the moral and ethical considerations that are so important for students participating in physical activity and leads to the opposite of the intended result—a population of inactive, disconnected students who see their sports-based programing as having little relevance to their own lives (Dyson, 2006; Gibbons, Wharf-Higgins, Gaul, & VanGyn, 1999; Humbert, 2006; Macdonald & Hunter, 2005). There is a need for a dialectical, reflexive process that reflects the characteristic of the social setting and the humanistic nature of the physical education environment. *Praxis* has these characteristics: "it remakes the conditions of informed action and constantly reviews action and the knowledge which informs it" (Carr & Kemmis, 1986, p. 33).

The concept of phronesis is more closely related to the principles of wisdom traditions because "the virtue associated with *praxis*, *phronesis*, concerns the affairs of human being" (Hanley, 1998, p. 4). Dunne (1993) further explains that phronesis is "personal knowledge in that, in the living of one's life, it characterizes and expresses the kind of person that one is" (p. 244). As Carson (2012) states, the "concept of *phronesis*, which relates to good character and ethical action in the service of the common good, may hold creative possibilities for a reinvigorated understanding of practice that is more appropriate to matters of human relationship" (p. 2).

As previously mentioned, phronesis "characterizes a person who knows how to live well (*eu zen*)" (Dunne, 1993, p. 244). For Kim, this wellness way of being a teacher is part of living in the tensionality of her pedagogical situation (Aoki, as cited in Pinar & Irwin, 2005). She responds to the lived situation moving beyond the technical rationality of implementation or "reproduc[-tion] of the curriculum-as-plan" (p. 162). She understands that she is not merely a "curriculum installer" and knows that how she does things comes from who she is, her being. This calls for embodied ways of knowing that draw on her empathy, kindness, and compassion—listening to her students as she is mindful that the students in front of her have lives of their own, requiring her to be attuned to the aliveness of each teaching situation. Working from within, Kim also knows teaching is "'a leading out to new possibilities,' to the 'not yet'" (p. 162). Her dialectical way of living curriculum with her students means she doesn't recognize a leader-follower action; she looks at pedagogic leading as "a responsible responding to students" (p. 213). This stems from her allowing herself to be vulnerable, letting go of her own attachments, living in the tensions, and indwelling between horizons of self/other, body/mind/spirit, theory/practice, curriculum-as-plan/curriculum-as-lived, well/unwell. This way of being a teacher is a pedagogical wisdom that is accompanied by an ontological "admission of the whole beings of teachers and students" (p. 245).

Understanding Students as Whole Beings

How can we ensure that children, as whole beings, remain at the core of the educational process? (Kumar, 2013). We are "living in an era of high-stakes accountability, standardized testing with a mechanistic consideration of students" (McClain, Ylimaki & Ford, 2010, p. 308) and with a "diminished attention to the whole child" (p. 308). Palmer (1993) warns, "when the life of the mind alienates more than it connects, the heart goes out of things, and there is little left to sustain us" (as cited in McClain, Ylimaki & Ford, 2010, p. 309). Kim has demonstrated that teaching with a wellness focus must begin with teachers' hearts opening to a vision of students' potential through creative exploration of all life forces and the balance of all the dimensions of the self (physical, emotional, spiritual, mental) so that children may subjectively come to know how to be whole (Hart, 2010).

It is even more important for physical education to consider a curriculum of wellness because the dominant discourse of how we view our students is rooted in Cartesian discourse where body and mind are separate. Tinning (1997) further explains,

> These are functionalist and foundationalist views of the body. The body is considered an object to be dissected, measured, probed, maintained, tuned, and compared. Our basic understandings of the body are embedded in the analogy of the body as a machine, an analogy that is reductionistic and mechanistic. (p. 107)

Other physical education scholars echo this view, as Bain (1990) explains, "consistent with technocratic ideology...a healthy body is often equated with performance or appearance" (p. 29). Further, many authors mention the "cult of the body" (Tinning & Glasby, 2002; Bain, 1990; Colquhoun, 1990; Tinning, 2004), which refers to the hegemony of physical appearance and performance as being a " signifier of worthiness" (Tinning & Glasby, 2002, p. 110). These authors also explain that despite research on the impact of how some cultural practices "contribute to limited, restricted or oppressive bodily practices, we have seen little significant systemic change" (Tinning, 2004, p. 219) in physical and health education.

Although much of pedagogical research in physical education still reinforces the cult of the body, the physical education community has discussed some alternative ways of understanding the body from a variety of philosophical perspectives. In a book chapter about the pedagogy of the body, Tinning (2010) presents different ways of thinking about the body, including: Zen body maintenance where exercise, spirituality and therapy are combined; the Alexander Technique that incorporates ideas of posture and conscious thought; somatic education; and sociological imagination that "challenges orthodoxy and provides the possibility of disrupting the cult of the body" (Tinning, 2010, p. 121).

Francis and Lu (2009) also highlight Eastern traditions in physical education and their potential to "promote body-mind unity, emphasize the process as well as the product; create a balance between the subjective experience and objective knowledge, and honor a harmonious relationship between humans and nature" (p. 23). Brown and Johnson (2000) outline the potential of martial arts as an Eastern movement form to enhance current practices in physical education that can help individuals in "adopting and integrating alternative philosophical outlooks toward life and physical activity" (p. 246). Part of the rationale for using these practices stems from the notion of balancing the more technocratic ways of physical education with a more "holistic self-development" approach grounded in axiological knowledge where aesthetics and morality in movement forms are embedded into the curriculum (Brown & Johnson, 2000).

Gerber and Morgan (1979) present perspectives that are contrary to the dualistic Cartesian way of thinking of the body: "the body is not an instrument of the mind nor is it connected to it.... The body is you; you are your body. Your body is your mode of being-in-the-world" (p. 146). This way of understanding the body is important to the field of physical education because there is a "lack of a presence in the discourse of physical education about the qualities and characteristics of the movement experience" (Brown & Payne, 2009, p. 418). Brown (2008) explains "lived bodily experiences are embodied and provide something more than just skill development, health or fitness" (p. 5).

It is clear that there is a need for input beyond the dominant collective identity to be able to understand students as whole beings, as the reductionistic tendencies to focus on the body are embedded in the life history of our field. Hence, the call to wisdom (Smith, 2013). Although already discussed in previous chapters, it is worth repeating here. One of the fundamental aspects of all wisdom traditions is that wellness is dependent upon unity within the self, between self and others (natural world and all living things), and between life and death. We have discussed how teachers' way of being—connected body, mind, and spirit—is essential to students being able to live healthfully—balanced wholeness and in harmony with the natural rhythms of the universe.

Examples of how unity, wholeness, balance, and harmony are understood and practiced are prominent throughout many of the wisdom traditions around the world. In Michael Hart's (1999) article, "Seeking Mino-pimatasiwin (the Good Life)," he explains the concept of wholeness through the medicine wheel (used by many Indigenous peoples such as Cree, Dakota, and Blackfoot), which is used to express relationships in sets of four, associated with the four cardinal directions: four aspects of humanness (emotional, physical, mental, spiritual), four cycles of life (birth/infancy, youth, adulthood, elder/death), four elements (fire, water, wind, earth), four seasons (spring, summer, fall, winter). Wholeness involves movement in/through all these aspects and is fundamental to the health of all living things. Of course, to move in this way one must recognize the need to balance our attention on the four aspects of these relationships so that one part is not emphasized at the detriment of the others. It is easy to see how other connections flow within and around these concepts such as harmony, growth (developing body, mind, spirit in harmony), and healing (restoring wholeness, balance).

In Daoism (Taoism), *qi* philosophy has a nondualistic perspective and considers *qi* the "principle of life." As such, "*qi* has the transformative power to turn our alienated perception of the objectivist consciousness (seeing things merely as objects) into animated perceptions that see the whole world as being suffused by a vital and sacred life force" (Bai & Cohen, 2008, p. 42). Not only is *qi* a "universal life principle," but it is also the foundation of being aware in the present moment (moment to moment) where an individual feels connected to everything/one in the world and universe. The embodiment of this philosophy requires sensing, feeling, seeing—with body, mind, spirit, and heart—in a way that harmonizes *qi* in the self with the universe into a whole. There are many Eastern practices, such as martial arts, qi gong, and calligraphy that work with the concept of qi (*ki* in Japanese). Furthermore, Buddhist, Zen Buddhist, and Confucian philosophies have a similar focus on the unity of self–other, subjective–objective, mind–body–spirit, where meditative practices, crafts, yoga, and Zen drawing are embodied to encourage living nondualistically and intersubjectively (Bai & Cohen, 2008).

While I am eager to share details of further practices that reflect wisdom's fundamental project, I am cautious that in doing so I may reinforce the commodified culture of wellness that seems to have manifested in the West. For example, through globalization, the world became familiar with yoga but very few *practice* yoga, which is the path that one can follow to achieve the spiritual goal of life (*Moksha, Samadhi,* or *Nirvana*). Hinduism is a wisdom tradition that is about a *Way* of life that considers the whole world as a single family that deifies the one truth and accepts all forms of beliefs. Hindu beliefs include Dharma (ethics/duties), Samsara (the continuing cycle of birth, life, death, and rebirth), Karma (action and subsequent reaction), Moksha (liberation from Samsara), and the various yogas (paths or practices) (Bhartiya Cultural Centre, 2010).

Much of the yoga "industry" seems to be marketed towards selling a product (classes, clothes, mats, etc.) and relaxation. I am questioning and pondering how this commodified culture follows yoga philosophy and what it has to do with living a *Way* of life. As a teacher who has attempted to "teach" yoga to high school students in a co-ed, multi-class environment, I completely missed the point that yoga is about *practicing* a Way to "live fully *in* the world in a healthy life-giving way" (Smith, 2011a, p. 172). My classes were often reduced to mere flexibility training sessions, missing the intended purpose of yoga.

Physical education's challenge is how to practice yoga and other traditions without it being a "prosthetic device" (Smith, 2011a, p. 172) to survive the challenges of putting up our education system as a product for sale. Helberg, Heyes, and Rohel (2009) explain how yoga can lead to students becoming better able to engage in movement in a mindful way and be reflective on embodied experiences, as well as being more present in movement—paying attention to the body's lived experience. There is value in teaching children the *practice* of yoga but within a curriculum of wellness with a grounding in wisdom that recognizes the subjective complexities of the tradition and focuses on how we live—interconnected, wholly, and ethically. This point can be extended to Kim's way of being a teacher, how she teaches, and the way she looks at her students. Again, it is about where you start. If it is from an objective position where the physical body (your own and your students') is an object, then you simply "apply" a strategy, activity, or exercise in a technical way that is removed from the subjectivity of the individual and realities of the world. However if you are focused on how you live your life as a teacher and seeing your students as whole beings, then the intent of these practices lies in "helping students recover the unity of their being" (Smith, 2011a, p. 175).

· 7 ·

A CURRICULUM OF WELLNESS

(RE)TURNING TO THE TREE(S)

I walk amongst the trees peering up into the sky, looking for
the compositions that excite my senses. I am filled with expectation, joy,
even laughter. There is such magic in the air.
— RITA IRWIN, 2006, P. 75

Somewhere along the way, the subjective attention and mindfulness I practiced in my childhood was moved to the background. I have already told
the story of my connection to a wonderful tree in our family orchard in the
Okanagan Valley, British Columbia, and my disconnection that subsequently
contributed to my own ill health in my adulthood. So, essentially my journey
to wisdom and a curriculum of wellness begins and continues with trees.

Let me be clear: trees are not just a root metaphor for my inquiry journey.
They are not just representations or models I wish to highlight to summarize
a theoretical underpinning to my work. The trees are living, breathing sen-
tient beings that had I not (re)connected with and continue to connect with,
I certainly would not be in my present location. The trees are a meditative
sensibility, and if I am not with, in, and around the trees, I am not present;
I do not feel whole. When I am with the trees I can (re)cover a sense of my
experiences growing up on a farm, I can feel the natural rhythms of the Earth.
I can be in the moment, each moment as if seeing it for the first time, every

time. It is here I am learning nonjudgment, patience, nonpermanence ("letting go"), trust, nonperfection, and acceptance.

Curriculum is about our lives and how we live them. The trees remind me that, as a person, a researcher, a teacher, teacher educator, I need to focus on the manner of living. The trees encourage the stillness that is needed to recover the mind–body–spirit connection that is critical to restoring balance and unity in ourselves and the world. If we pay attention, the trees are prompting us to challenge our assumptions about how we conduct ourselves in this world, to "see" the real origins of our problems, to name our struggles for what they are. I listen to the trees as they tell stories of all the other relationships they have with the sun, moon, earth, water, animals (two-legged, four-legged, winged, crawling), and plants—relationships that are reciprocal and essential to the health of the planet. When I am in stillness with a tree or trees, I feel the energy flow of the universe and I have an aesthetic awareness of my connection to all living things.

The trees have helped restore my view, my passion, and my vision for the future in physical education—to what is not yet. I acknowledge that some of my writing may seem critical of myself and the field, but these are the moments of progression and regression that I have illuminated to form the present that have helped me to truly see what is actually in front of us, individually and collectively. It is true that there are a variety of views about physical education that are living within classrooms on this planet and I am now open to seeing those (multiple) perspectives and thus better able to synthesize each present moment as a situated individual connected to others.

My final point is that without (re)turning to the trees, living this type of inquiry would not have been possible for me. It is not about the trees themselves but my connection to the trees where I am able to feel strength and balance—physically, emotionally, mentally, and spiritually. This is my practice of mindfulness—paying attention to the whole person, the whole forest *and* the one tree. Kabat-Zinn (1994) explains that wholeness "is always within us, usually as a vague feeling or memory left over from when we were children" (p. 95). Mindful practice reminds us that we are already whole.

This mindful practice is not a specific place I go to practice some technical skills to achieve a goal (as was my life as an athlete, coach, and physical educator). This is a way of life, a way of being that nurtures individual and collective wellness. My dynamic active journey, your journey, our collective journeys in the circle of life are full of pedagogical moments for us to pay attention to—this is curriculum. And teaching *a curriculum of wellness* is living life in this way.

This is my *present* location and synthetical *moment* of inquiry.

NOTES

Introduction

1. In bracketing "physical," I am merely suggesting that this conversation can be applied to the broader educational environment. Much of what is presented in this book involves what it means to teach a curriculum of wellness, and this can take place in any classroom, school, community, or home around the world.

2. The term *currere* is the Latin infinitive of "curriculum," which means "the running of the course" (curriculum, n.d.). *Currere* is theoretically grounded in existentialism, phenomenology, and psychoanalysis, and emphasizes the active nature of curriculum. The method of *currere* is an autobiographical process for individuals to "sketch the relations among school knowledge, life history, and intellectual development in ways that might function self-transformatively" (Pinar, Reynolds, Slattery & Taubman, 1995, p. 515).

3. This inquiry process relied upon a collaborative, reciprocal, and democratic relationship between the teacher-participant and researcher. This type of research is done *with* instead of *on* the teacher, where decision making is a shared process and meaning is co-generated.

4. Nonduality refers to unity rather than separateness. Nondualistic thinking rejects the subject-object dichotomy that is historically rooted in Plato's dichotomy of Being and Becoming, Kant's phenomenal mental world and noumenal material world, and Descartes' body-mind dualism where mental substance (thinking) and corporeal substance (physical dimension) are separate entities (also known as Cartesian dualism). Rejecting the body-mind dualism allows us to consider the "embodied persons' subjective experience in the world" (Rintala, 1991, p. 274).

5. The meaning of health is *whole*. As Kabat-Zinn (1990) explains, "whole implies integration, an interconnectedness of all parts…the nature of wholeness is that it is always present" (p. 162) and embedded in a larger wholeness. Health then is a "dynamic process, an inner balancing with our self and the universe. We may experience distortions, distractions, illness, and this disrupts our inner balance and constantly undermines experiencing our intrinsic wholeness" (p. 164). This will be further explored in subsequent chapters.

6. Pinar (2004) believes that "the complicated conversation that is the curriculum requires interdisciplinary intellectuality, erudition, and self-reflexivity" (p. 8). In his discussion about the anti-intellectualism in the field of education, Pinar (2004) encourages the profession to "engage in 'complicated conversation' with our subject, our students, and ourselves" (p. 9). Further reference to Pinar's (2004) notion of a "complicated conversation" will be represented in italicized text.

Chapter 1

1. Doerr (2004) also reminds us that because *currere* is a dynamic and active process and we are always responding to experiences, "there is never a finale; the work is constantly in process" (p. 184). Kim and I understood that as we moved through the semester our analysis would produce new insights and synthetical moments, allowing for a deeper meaning and understanding about a curriculum of wellness. The end point to our particular inquiry process was a function of the school system's timeline of a semester but it should be noted that the *currere* process in relation to the course continues for both of us today.

2. These concepts will be further developed in the next chapter that outlines the theoretical framework for this inquiry.

3. Examples of other philosophers who have further explored the relationship between technical and practical reason include Newman, Collingwood, Arendt, Gadamer, Habermas, and Heidegger.

4. Generally, I am organizing knowledge in the philosophical categories of: epistemology (knowledge), axiology (values, ethics), ontology (being), and cosmology (universe, cosmos).

Chapter 2

1. The author makes a special note of the spelling of *wholistic*: "This spelling is used to represent the meaning of the 'whole.' The more common spelling, holistic, leaves the impression of something that has a void" (p. 18).

Chapter 4

1. Georgette Reed is the head coach of the University of Alberta Track, Field and Cross Country program. Georgette represented Canada in shot put in various international

events including the Olympic Games and Commonwealth Games. Prior to her track and field successes, Georgette was a swimmer for Washington State University but consistent overtraining and ongoing rotator cuff injuries ended her swimming career. She is frequently asked as a guest speaker at schools and events to share her struggles about her life as a student, athlete, and coach, and how she overcame these challenges.

Chapter 5

1. Yoga Nidra, also known as sleep with awareness, is a practice that promotes full-body relaxation and a deep meditative state. Typically it includes a guided body scan through verbal cues. It is different from Savasana at the end of a yoga session, as more time is spent to address physiological and spiritual needs (Levin-Gervasi, 2007).

BIBLIOGRAPHY

Active Healthy Kids Canada. (2014). *Active Healthy Kids Canada report card on physical activity for children and youth*. Retrieved from http://www.participaction.com/wp-content/uploads/2015/03/AHKC_2014_ReportCard_ENG.pdf

Adelman, C. (1993). Kurt Lewin and the origins of action research. *Educational Action Research, 1*(1), 7–24.

Alberta Education. (2000). *K–12 physical education: Guide to implementation*. Edmonton: Alberta Education.

Alberta Education. (2008). *Wellness curricula to improve the health of children and youth: A review and synthesis of related literature*. Edmonton: Alberta Education.

Alberta Education. (2009). *Framework for kindergarten to grade 12 wellness education*. Edmonton: Alberta Education.

Alberta Education. (2013). Statistics: Education facts, rates and demographic information. Retrieved from http://education.alberta.ca/department/stats.aspx

Alberta Teachers' Association. (2000). *Action research guide for Alberta teachers*. Edmonton, Alberta: Alberta Teachers' Association.

Altrichter, H., Kemmis, S., McTaggart, R., & Zuber-Skerritt, O. (2002). The concept of action research. *The Learning Organization, 9*(3), 125–131.

Aoki, T. (2005). Teaching as indwelling between two curriculum worlds (1986/1991). In W. Pinar & R. Irwin (Eds.), *Curriculum in a new key: The collected works of Ted. T. Aoki* (pp. 159–165). Mahwah, NJ: Lawrence Erlbaum.

APPLE Schools. (2013). Alberta project promoting active living and healthy eating. Retrieved from http://www.appleschools.ca

Archibald, J. (2008). *Indigenous storywork: Educating the heart, mind, body, and spirit*. Vancouver: UBC Press.

Armour, K. (2006). The way to a teacher's heart: Narrative research in physical education. In D. Kirk, D. Macdonald, & M. O'Sullivan (Eds.), *The physical education handbook* (pp. 467–485). Thousand Oaks, CA: Sage.

Arnold (1979). *Meaning in movement, sport and physical education*. London: Heinemann.

Bai, H. (2001). Beyond the educated mind: Towards a pedagogy of mindfulness. In B. Hockings, J. Haskell, & W. Linds (Eds.), *Unfolding bodymind: Exploring possibilities through education* (pp. 86–99). Brandon, VT: Foundation for Educational Renewal.

Bai & Cohen (2008). Breathing Qi (Ch'i), following Dao (Tao): Transforming this violence-ridden world. In C. Eppert, & H. Wang (Eds.), *Cross-cultural studies in curriculum: Eastern thought, educational insights* (pp. 35–54). New York, NY: Taylor & Francis.

Bain, L. (1990). A critical analysis of the hidden curriculum in physical education. In D. Kirk & R. Tinning (Eds.), *Physical education curriculum and culture: Critical issues in the contemporary crisis* (pp. 23–42). London: Falmer Press.

Bain, L. (1995). Mindfulness and subjective knowledge. *Quest, 47*(2), 239–253.

Basso, K. (1996). *Wisdom sits in places: Landscape and language among the Western Apache*. Albuquerque: University of New Mexico Press.

Beck, C. (1993). *Nothing special: Living Zen*. New York, NY: Harper.

Bhartiya Cultural Centre. (2010). *Beliefs*. Edmonton: Bhartiya Cultural Society of Alberta. Retrieved from edmontonmandir.com

Bourdieu, P. (1998, December). The essence of neoliberalism. *Le Monde Diplomatique*. Retrieved from http://mondediplo.com/1998/12/08bourdieu

Boyce, W., King, M., & Roche, J. (2008). *Healthy settings for young people in Canada*. Public Health Agency of Canada. Retrieved from http://publications.gc.ca/collections /collection_2008/phac-aspc/HP35-6-2007E.pdf

Bradley, J., & Mackinlay, E. (2007). Singing the land, singing the family: Song, place and spirituality amongst the Yanyuwa. In F. Richards (Ed.), *The soundscapes of Australia: Music, place and spirituality* (pp. 75–92). Aldershot, UK: Ashgate.

Britzman, D. (1991). *Practice makes practice*. Albany: State University of New York Press.

Brown, D. (2007). *Restorying ourselves: Using currere to examine teachers' careers*. (Doctoral dissertation). Retrieved from http://digital.library.okstate.edu/etd/umi-okstate-2383.pdf

Brown, D., & Johnson, A. (2000). The social practice of self-defense martial arts: Application for physical education. *Quest, 52*(3), 246–259.

Brown, T. (2008). Movement and meaning-making in physical education. *ACHPER Healthy Lifestyles Journal, 55*(2/3), 5–9.

Brown, T., & Payne, P. (2009). Conceptualizing the phenomenology of movement in physical education: Implications for pedagogic inquiry and development. *Quest, 61*, 418–441.

Butler, J. (2006). Curriculum constructions of ability: Enhancing learning through Teaching Games for Understanding (TGfU) as a curriculum model. *Sport, Education and Society, 11*(3), 243–258.

Butler, M. (2011). *Introduction to Buddhism*. Retrieved from http://www.buddhanet.net/e-learning/intro_bud.htm

Cale, L., & Harris, J. (2009). Fitness testing in physical education—a misdirected effort in promoting healthy lifestyles and physical activity? *Physical Education and Sport Pedagogy*, *14*(1), 89–108.

Canadian Mental Health Association, Alberta Division. (2011). Mental illness in Canada. Retrieved from http://www.cmha.ab.ca/bins/ site_page.asp?cid=284-285-1258-1404& lang=1#6

Carr, W., & Kemmis, S. (1986). *Becoming critical: Education, knowledge and action research*. Philadelphia: Falmer Press.

Carr, W., & Kemmis, S. (2009). Educational action research: A critical approach. In S. Noffke & B. Somekh (Eds.), *The Sage handbook of educational action research* (pp. 74–84). London, UK: Sage

Carson, T. (2012). Remembering ethics: Fostering practical reason in an age of science. In D. E. Lund, L. Panayotidis, H. Smits, & J. Towers (Eds.), *Provoking conversations on inquiry in teacher education*. New York, NY: Peter Lang.

Casey, E. (1996). How to get from space to place in a fairly short stretch of time. In S. Feld & K. Basso (Eds.), *Senses of place*, (pp. 13–52). Santa Fe, NM: School of American Research Press.

Chodron, P. (1994). *Start where you are: A guide to compassionate living*. Boston: Shambhala.

Cohen, A., & Bai, H. (2007). Dao and Zen of teaching: Classroom as enlightenment field. *Educational Insights*, *11*(3), 1–14.

Colquhoun, D. (1990). Images of healthism in health-based physical education. In D. Kirk & R. Tinning (Eds.), *Physical education curriculum and culture: Critical issues in the contemporary crisis* (pp. 225–251). London, UK: Falmer Press.

Confuscianism. (n.d.). Confucianism. Retrieved from http://confucianism. freehostingguru. com/

Craig, R., et al. (2009). *Health Survey for England 2008. Physical activity and fitness*. Leeds, UK: The NHS Information Centre for Health and Social Care. Retrieved from http://www. hscic.gov.uk/pubs/hse08physicalactivity

Creswell, J. (2005). *Educational research: Planning, conducting, and evaluating quantitative and qualitative research* (2nd ed.). Upper Saddle River, NJ: Pearson.

Csikszentmihalyi, M. (1997). *Finding flow: The psychology of engagement with everyday life*. New York, NY: Basic Books.

Curriculum. (n.d.). Online etymology dictionary. Retrieved from http://www.etymonline.com/ index.php?term=curriculum&allowed_in_frame=0

Dalai Lama. (2001). *Ethics for the new millennium*. New York, NY: Riverhead Books.

Dale, R. (2006). *The Tao Te Ching: A new translation, commentary and introduction*. London: Watkins.

David Suzuki Foundation. (2010). *The "dirty dozen" ingredients investigated in the David Suzuki Foundation survey of chemicals in cosmetics*. Retrieved from http://www.davidsuzuki.org/issues/downloads/Dirty-dozen-backgrounder.pdf

Dentro, K., et al. (2014). Results from the United States 2014 report card on physical activity for children and youth. *Journal of Physical Activity and Health*, *11* (Supp. 1), S105–S112.

Devis-Devis, J. (2006). Socially critical research perspectives in physical education. In D. Kirk, D. Macdonald & M. O'Sullivan (Eds.), *The physical education handbook* (pp. 37–58). Thousand Oaks, CA: Sage.

Devis-Devis, J., & Sparkes, A. (1999). Burning the book: A biographical study of a pedagogically inspired identity crisis in physical education. *European Physical Education Review*, 5(2), 135–152.

Dietary Guidelines Advisory Committee. (2010). *Report of the Dietary Guidelines Advisory Committee on the Dietary Guidelines for Americans, 2010, to the Secretary of Agriculture and the Secretary of Health and Human Services.* Washington, DC: U.S. Department of Agriculture.

Doerr, M. (2004). *Currere and the environmental autobiography.* New York, NY: Peter Lang.

Donald, D. (2011). EDSE 504 Curriculum inquiry. (Unpublished course syllabus). Edmonton: University of Alberta.

Dunne, J. (1993). *Back to the rough ground: "Phronesis" and "techne" in modern philosophy and in Aristotle.* Notre Dame, IN: University of Notre Dame Press.

Dyson, B. (2006). Students' perspectives of physical education. In D. Kirk, D. Macdonald, & M. O'Sullivan (Eds.), *The handbook of physical education* (pp. 326–346). Thousand Oaks, CA: Sage.

Elliott, J. (1991). *Action research for educational change.* Milton Keynes, PA: Open University Press.

Eppert, C., & Wang, H. (2008). *Cross-cultural studies in curriculum: Eastern thought, educational insights.* New York, NY: Taylor & Francis.

Ethos. (n.d.). Online etymology dictionary. Retrieved from http://www.etymonline.com/index.php?allowed_in_frame=0&search=ethos&searchmode=none

Evans, J. (2004) Making a difference? Education and "ability" in physical education, *European Physical Education Review*, 10(1), 95–108.

Ever Active Schools. (n.d.). Ever active schools.. Retrieved from http://www.everactive.org

Feldman, A. (2002). Existential approaches to action research. *Educational Action Research*, 10(2), 233–252.

Feldman, A. (2009). Existentialism and action research. In S. Noffke & B. Somekh (Eds.), *Sage handbook of educational action research* (pp. 381–391). London, UK: Sage.

Fernandez-Balboa, J. (1997). *Critical postmodernism in human movement, physical education, and sport.* Albany: State University of New York Press.

Fitzclarence, L., & Tinning, R. (1990). Challenging hegemonic physical education: Contextualizing physical education as an examinable subject. In D. Kirk & R. Tinning (Eds.), *Physical education curriculum and culture: Critical issues in the contemporary crisis* (pp. 169–192). London, UK: Falmer Press.

Fowler, L. (2006). *A curriculum of difficulty: Narrative research in education and the practice of teaching.* New York, NY: Peter Lang.

Francis, N., & Lu, C. (2009). The conceptual framework of the Eastern approach in physical education: Ancient wisdom for modern times. *ACHPER Healthy Lifestyle Journal*, 5(2), 23–27.

Gerber, E. W., & Morgan, W. J. (Eds.) (1979). *Sport and the body: A philosophical symposium* (2nd ed.). Philadelphia, PA: Lea & Febiger.

Gibbons, S., & Gaul, C. (2004). Making physical education meaningful for young women: Case study in educational change. *Avante, 10*(2), 1–16.

Gibbons, S., Wharf-Higgins, J., Gaul, C., & VanGyn, G. (1999). Listening to female students in high school physical education. *Avante, 5*(2), 1–20.

Giroux, H., Penna, A., & Pinar, W. (Eds.) (1981). *Curriculum and instruction: Alternatives in education.* Berkeley, CA: McCutchan.

Goodson, I. (1997). *The changing curriculum: Studies in social construction.* New York, NY: Peter Lang.

Graham, R. (1992). Currere and reconceptualism: The progress of the pilgrimage 1975–1990. *Journal of Curriculum Studies, 24*(1), 27–42.

Greene, M. (1971). Curriculum and consciousness. In D. Flinders & S. Thornton (Eds.) *The curriculum studies reader* (2004, pp. 135–148). New York, NY: Falmer.

Greene, M. (1973). *Teacher as stranger: Educational philosophy for the modern age.* Belmont, CA: Wadsworth.

Greene, M. (1977). Toward wide-awakeness: An argument for the arts and humanities in education. *Teachers College Record, 79*(1), 119–125.

Greene, M. (1978). *Landscapes of Learning.* New York, NY: Teachers College Press.

Greene, M. (1984a). "Excellence," meanings, and multiplicity. *Teachers College Record, 86*(2), 283–297.

Greene, M. (1984b). How do we think about our craft? *Teachers College Record, 86*(1), 55–67.

Greene, M. (1988). *The dialectic of freedom.* New York, NY: Teachers College Press.

Greene, M. (1996). I am not yet. In W. Pinar, *Intellectual advancement through disciplinarity: Verticality and horizontality in curriculum studies* (2007, pp. 151–156). Rotterdam, Netherlands: Sense.

Greenwood, D., & Levin, M. (2007). *Introduction to action research: Social research for social change.* Thousand Oaks, CA: Sage.

Grumet, M. (1980). Autobiography and reconceptualization. In W. Pinar (Ed.), *Contemporary curriculum discourses: Twenty years of JCT* (pp. 24–29). New York, NY: Peter Lang.

Grumet, M. (1987). The politics of personal knowledge. *Curriculum Inquiry, 17*(3), 319–329.

Grumet, M. R. (1988). *Bitter milk: Women and teaching.* Amherst: University of Massachusetts Press.

Halas, J. (2002). Engaging alienated youth in physical education: An alternative program with lessons for the traditional class. *Journal of Teaching in Physical Education, 21,* 267–286.

Halas, J. (2011). Aboriginal youth and their experiences in physical education: "This is what you taught me." *PHENex Journal, 3*(2), 1–23.

Hanley. C. (1998, August). *Theory and praxis in Aristotle and Heidegger.* Paper presented at the Twentieth World Congress of Philosophy, Boston MA. Retrieved from http://www.bu.edu/wcp/Papers/Acti/ActiHanl.htm

Hardman, K. (2008). The situation of physical education in schools: A European perspective. *Human Movement, 9*(1), 5–18.

Hardman, K. (2013). Global issues in physical education: Worldwide physical education survey III findings. *International Journal of Physical Education, 50*(3), 15–28.

Hardman, K., & Marshall, J. (2000). The state and status of physical education in schools in the international context. *European Physical Education Review, 6*(3), 203–229.

Hardman, K., & Marshall, J. (2005). *Update on the state and status of physical education worldwide.* International Council of Sport and Physical Education 2nd World Summit on Physical Education, Switzerland. Retrieved from http://www.icsspe.org/content/2nd-world-summit-physical-education-0

Harris, J., & Cale, L. (2007). Physical education and childhood obesity. *Physical Education Matters, 2*(4), 10–14.

Hart, M. A. (1999). Seeking mino-pimatasiwin (the good life): An Aboriginal approach to social work practice. *Native Social Work Journal, 2*(1), 91–112.

Hart, M. A. (2008). Critical reflections on an aboriginal approach to helping. In M. Gray, J. Coates, & M. Yellow Bird (Eds.), *Indigenous social work around the world: Towards culturally relevant education and practice* (pp. 59–70). Burlington, VT: Ashgate.

Hart, M. A. (2010) Indigenous worldviews, knowledge, and research: The development of an Indigenous research paradigm. *Journal of Indigenous Voices in Social Work, 1*(1), 1–16.

Hartke, J. (1990). Introduction. In E. McGaa, *Mother Earth spirituality: Native American paths to healing ourselves and our world* (pp. xiii–xviii). San Francisco, CA: Harper.

health. (n.d.). Online etymology dictionary. Retrieved from http://www.etymonline com/index.php?search=health&searchmode=none

Helberg, N., Heyes, C., & Rohel, J. (2009). Thinking through the body: Yoga, philosophy, and physical education. *Teaching Philosophy, 32*(3), 263–284.

Hellison, D, (1985). *Goals and strategies for teaching physical education.* Champaign, IL: Human Kinetics.

Hellison, D. (2011). *Teaching personal and social responsibility through physical activity.* Champaign, IL: Human Kinetics.

Herr, K., & Anderson, G. (2005). *The action research dissertation: A guide for students and faculty.* Thousand Oaks, CA: Sage.

Hill, D. (2009). Traditional medicine and restoration of wellness strategies. *Journal of Aboriginal Health, 5*(1), 26–42.

Humbert, L. (2005). Carpe diem: A challenge for us all. *Physical and Health Education, 71*(3), 4–13.

Humbert, L. (2006). Listening for a change: Understanding the experiences of students in physical education. In E. Singleton & A. Varpalotai (Eds.), *Stones in the sneaker: Active theory for secondary school physical and health educators* (pp. 155–181). London, ON: Althouse.

Hunter, L. (2006). Pleasure or pain: Student's perspectives on HPE. In R. Tinning and L. Hunter (Eds.), *Teaching health and physical education in Australian schools* (pp. 127–133). Melbourne, Australia: Pearson.

inquire. (n.d.). Online etymology dictionary. Retrieved from http://www.etymonline.com/index.php?allowed_in_frame=0&search=inquire&searchmode=none

International Union for Health Promotion and Education (IUHPE). (2010). *Promoting health in schools: From evidence to action.* Saint Denis, France: IUHPE.

Irwin, R. (2006). Walking to create an aesthetic and spiritual currere. *Visual Arts Research, 32*(1), 75–82.

Jamieson, R. (2011, February 18). Indigenous wisdom and geopolitics. *Global Brief.* Retrieved from http://globalbrief.ca/blog/2011/02/18/ nature-spirituality-and-politics-indigenous-wisdom-for-the-new-century/

Janssen, I., et al. (2004). Overweight and obesity in Canadian adolescents and their associations with dietary habits and physical activity patterns. *Journal of Adolescent Health, 35*(5), 360–367.

Jewett, A., & Bain, L. (1985). *The curriculum process in physical education.* Dubuque, IA: Wm. C. Brown.

Jewett, A., Bain, L., & Ennis, C. (1995). *The curriculum process in physical education* (2nd ed.). Madison, WI: Brown & Benchmark.

Jewett, A., & Mullan, M. (1977). *Curriculum design: Purposes and processes in physical education teaching-learning.* Washington, DC: American Association of Health, Physical Education, and Recreation.

Joint Consortium for School Health. (n.d.). What is a "comprehensive school health approach"? *JCSH.* Retrieved from http://www.jcsh-cces.ca/index.php/about/comprehensive-school-health/what-is-csh

Kabat-Zinn, J. (1990). *Full catastrophe living.* New York, NY: Random House.

Kabat-Zinn, J. (1994). *Wherever you go, there you are.* New York, NY: Hyperion.

Kalyn, B. (2006). *A healthy journey: Indigenous teachings that direct culturally responsive curricula in physical education.* (Unpublished doctoral dissertation.) University of Alberta, Edmonton.

Kemmis, S., & McTaggart, R. (1988). Introduction: The nature of action research. In S. Kemmis & R. McTaggart (Eds.), *The action research planner* (3rd ed.) (pp. 5–28). Geelong, Victoria, Australis: Deakin University Press.

Kilborn, M.(1999). *Investigating female student enrollment in physical education 11.* (Unpublished master's thesis.) University of Victoria, Victoria, BC.

Kilborn, M. (2011). *Physical education curriculum across Canada.* Presentation at the Canadian Society for the Study of Education Conference, Fredericton, NB.

Kilborn, M., Lorusso, J., & Francis, N. (2015). An analysis of Canadian physical education curricula. *European Physical Education Review.* Advance online publication. doi: 10.1177/1356336X15586909

Kirby, A. (2007). A qualitative investigation of physical activity challenges and opportunities in a northern-rural Aboriginal community: Voices from within. *Pimatisiwin: A Journal of Aboriginal & Indigenous Community Health, 5*(1), 5–24.

Kirk, D. (1988). *Physical education and curriculum study: A critical introduction.* London, UK: Croom Helm.

Kirk, D. (1993). Curriculum work in physical education: Beyond the objectives approach? *Journal of Teaching in Physical Education, 12,* 244–265.

Kirk, D. (1998). *Schooling bodies: School practice and public discourse 1880–1950*. London, UK: Leicester University Press.

Kirk, D. (2010). *Physical education futures*. London, UK: Routledge.

Kirk, D. (2013). Physical education for the 21st century. In S. Capel & M. Whitehead (Eds.), *Debates in physical education*. London, UK: Routledge.

Kornfield, J. (2000). *After the ecstasy, the laundry: How the heart grows wise on the spiritual path*. New York, NY: Bantam Books.

Kumar, A. (2013). *Curriculum as meditative inquiry*. New York, NY: Palgrave Macmillan.

Kuyvenhoven, J. (2005). *In the presence of each other: A pedagogy of storytelling*. (Unpublished doctoral dissertation.) University of British Columbia, Vancouver, BC.

Kwan, T. (2008). The overdominance of English in global education: Is an alternative scenario thinkable? In R. Ames & P. Hershock (Eds.), *Educations and their purposes: A conversation among cultures* (pp. 54–71). Honolulu: University of Hawaii Press.

Lai, C. (2008). The ideas of "educating" and "learning" in Confucian thought. In R. Ames & P. Hershock (Eds.), *Educations and their purposes: A conversation among cultures* (pp. 310–326). Honolulu: University of Hawaii Press.

Lawson, H. (2009). Paradigms, exemplars and social change. *Sport, Education and Society, 14*, 77–100.

Levin-Gervasi, S. (2007, August). Find full-body relaxation in yoga nidra. *Yoga Journal*. Retrieved from http://www.yogajournal.com/article/health/in-need-of-yoga-nidra/

Lewin, K. (1946). Action research and minority problems. *Journal of Social Issues, 2*(4), 34–46.

life. (n.d.). Online etymology dictionary. Retrieved from http://www.etymonline.com/index.php?allowed_in_frame=0&search=life&searchmode=none

Lincoln, Y., & Guba, E. (1985). *Naturalistic inquiry*. Los Angeles, CA: Sage.

Lloyd, R. (2011). Awakening movement consciousness in the physical landscapes of literacy: Leaving, reading and being moved by one's trace. *Phenomenology and Practice, 5*(2), 70–92.

Lloyd, R., & Smith, S. (2009, December). Enlivening the curriculum of health-related fitness. *Educational Insights, 13*(4).

Locke, L. (1992). Changing secondary school physical education. *Quest, 44*, 361–372.

Lodewyk, K., Lu, C., & Kentel, J. (2009). Enacting the spiritual dimension in physical education. *Physical Educator, 66*(4), 170.

Lu, C., Tito, J., & Kentel, J. (2009). Eastern movement disciplines (EMDs) and mindfulness: A new path to subjective knowledge in Western physical education. *Quest, 63*, 353–369.

Lund, J., & Tannehill, D. (2005). Building a quality physical education program. In J. Lund & D. Tannehill (Eds.), *Standards-based physical education curriculum development* (pp. 16–46). Sudbury, MA: Jones and Bartlett.

Macdonald, D., & Hunter, L. (2005). Lessons learned…about curriculum: Five years on and half a world away. *Journal of Teaching in Physical Education, 24*, 111–126.

Macdonald, D., Kirk, D., Metzler, M., Nilges, L., Schempp, P., & Wright, J. (2002). It's all very well, in theory: Theoretical perspectives and their applications in contemporary pedagogical research. In R. Bailey & D. Kirk (Eds.), *Routledge physical education reader*, (pp. 369–392). London, UK: Routledge.

Maivorsdotter, N., & Lundvall, S. (2009). Aesthetic experience as an aspect of embodied learning: Stories from physical education student teachers. *Sport, Education and Society, 14*(3), 265–279.

Markula, P. (2004). Embodied movement knowledge in fitness and exercise education. In L. Bresler (Ed.), *Knowing bodies, moving minds: Towards embodied teaching and learning* (pp. 61–76). Dordrecht, Netherlands: Kluwer Academic.

McClain, L., Ylimaki, R., & Ford, M. (2010). Sustaining the heart of education: Finding space for wisdom and compassion. *International Journal of Children's Spirituality, 15*(4), 307–316.

McCuaig, L. (2006). HPE in the health promoting school. In R. Tinning, L. McCuaig, & L. Hunter (Eds.), *Teaching health and physical education in Australian schools* (pp. 56–69). Melbourne, Australia: Pearson.

McCuaig & Hay (2012). Principled pursuits of "the good citizen" in health and physical education. *Physical Education and Sport Pedagogy, 18*(3), 282–297.

McCuaig, L., Quennerstedt, M., & Macdonald, D. (2013). A salutogenic, strengths-based approach as a theory to guide HPE curriculum change. *Asia-Pacific Journal of Health, Sport and Physical Education, 4*(2).

McKernan, J. (1996). *Curriculum action research: A handbook of methods and resources for the reflective practitioner* (2nd ed.). London, UK: Kogan Page.

Mehl-Madrona, L. (2005). *Coyote wisdom: The power of story in healing.* Rochester, VT: Bear & Company.

Meili, D. (1991). *Those who know: Profiles of Alberta's Native Elders.* Edmonton, AB: NeWest Press.

Metzler, M. (2005). *Instructional models for physical education* (2nd ed.). Scottsdale, AZ: Holcomb Hathaway.

Nhat Hanh, T. (1987). *Being peace.* Berkeley, CA: Parallax Press.

Noffke, S. (2009). Revisiting the professional, personal, and political dimensions of action research. In S. Noffke & B. Somekh (Eds.), *The Sage handbook of educational action research* (pp. 6–23), Thousand Oaks, CA: Sage.

Oakley, S. (2011). *Black Plume's Blackfeet.* Retrieved from http://www.angelfire.com/stars4/blackfeetdanceman/BlackPlumeFrontPage.html

Ogden, C. L., Carroll, M. D., Kit, B. K., & Flegal, K. M. (2014, February 26). Prevalence of childhood and adult obesity in the United States, 2011–2012. *Journal of the American Medical Association, 311*(8), 806–814. Retrieved from http://jama.jamanetwork.com/article.aspx?articleid=1832542

Ovens, A., & Fletcher, T. (2014). *Self-study in physical education teacher education: Exploring the interplay of practice and scholarship.* New York, NY: Springer.

Park, O. (1996). *An invitation to dialogue between East and West: A critique of the modern and the post-modern thought.* New York, NY: Peter Lang.

Park, S. (2007). Enacting a "curriculum of life": Mindfulness and complexity thinking in the classroom. *Paideusis, 16*(3), 45–55.

Patel, R. (2009). *The value of nothing: Why everything costs so much more than we think.* Toronto, ON: HarperCollins.

Pautz, A. (1998). Views across the expanse: Maxine Greene's landscapes of learning. In W. Pinar (Ed.), *The passionate mind of Maxine Greene*. Bristol, PA: Falmer.

Perou, R., et al. (2013). Mental health surveillance among children—United States, 2005–2011. *Morbidity and Mortality Weekly Report, 67*(2), 1–35. Retrieved from http://www.cdc.gov/mmwr/preview/mmwrhtml/su6202a1.htm

Pewewardy, C. (1999, Autumn). The holistic medicine wheel. An Indigenous model of teaching and learning. *Winds of Change*, 28–31.

Pinar, W. (1975). Search for a method. In W. Pinar (Ed.), *Curriculum theorizing: The reconceptualists* (pp. 415–424). Berkeley, CA: McCutchan.

Pinar, W. (1978/2004). The reconceptualization of curriculum studies. In D. Hinders & S. Thornton (Eds.), *The curriculum studies reader* (2nd ed.) (pp. 149–157). New York, NY: Routledge.

Pinar, W. F. (1994). *Autobiography, politics and sexuality: Essays in curriculum theory 1972–1992*. New York, NY: Peter Lang.

Pinar, W. (2004). *What is curriculum theory?* Mahwah, NJ: Lawrence Erlbaum.

Pinar, W. (2007). *Intellectual advancement through disciplinarity: Verticality and horizontality in curriculum studies*. Rotterdam, Netherlands: Sense.

Pinar, W. (2012). *What is curriculum theory?* (2nded.). New York, NY: Routledge.

Pinar, W., & Grumet, M. (1976). *Toward a poor curriculum*. Dubuque, IA: Kendall/Hunt.

Pinar, W., & Irwin, R. (2005). *Curriculum in a new key: The collected works of Ted T. Aoki*. Mahwah, NJ: Lawrence Erlbaum.

Pinar, W., Reynolds, W., Slattery, P., & Taubman, P. (2004). *Understanding curriculum*. New York, NY: Peter Lang.

Plotnikoff, R., et al. (2009). Chronic disease-related lifestyle risk factors in a sample of Canadian adolescents. *Journal of Adolescent Health, 44* (6), 606–609.

Poonamallee, L. (2009). Building grounded theory in action research through the interplay of subjective ontology and objective epistemology. *Action Research, 7*(1), 69–83.

Rink, J. (1985). *Teaching physical education for learning*. St. Louis, MO: Times Mirror/ Mosby.

Rintala, J. (1991). The mind-body revisited. *Quest, 43*, 260–279.

Roberts, K., & Danoff-Burg, S. (2010). Mindfulness and health behaviors: Is paying attention good for you? *Journal of American College Health, 59*(3), 165–173.

Robinson, D. (1990). Wisdom through the ages. In R. Sternberg (Ed), *Wisdom: Its nature, origins and development* (pp. 13–24). New York, NY: Cambridge University Press.

Robinson, K. (2008). Changing paradigms. RSA. Retrieved from https://www.thersa.org/discover/videos/event-videos/2008/06/changing-paradigms/

Safrit, M. (1990). The validity and reliability of fitness tests for children: A review. *Pediatric Exercise Science, 2*, 9–28.

Salmon, E. (2000). Kincentric ecology: Indigenous perceptions of the human-nature relationship. *Ecological Applications, 10*(5), 1327–1332.

Salter, G. (2000). Marginalising Indigenous knowledge in teaching physical education: The sanitizing of hauora (wellbeing) in the new HPE curriculum. *Journal of Physical Education in New Zealand, 33*(1), 5–16.

Schaefer, L. (2013). Beginning teacher attrition: A question of identity making and identity shifting. *Teachers and Teaching: Theory and Practice, 19*(3), 260–274.

Schranz, N., et al. (2014). Results from Australia's 2014 report card on physical activity for children and youth. *Journal of Physical Activity and Health, 11*(Supp. 1), S1–S25.

Schubert, W. (2009). *Currere* and disciplinarity in curriculum studies: Possibilities for education research. *Educational Researcher, 38*(2), 136–140.

Share the World's Resources. (2010, November 17). *The Wisdom of Indigenous Cultures.* Retrieved from http://www.sharing.org/information-centre/articles/wisdom-indigenous-cultures

Siedentop, D., Mand, C., & Taggart, A. (1986). *Physical education: Teaching and curriculum strategies for grades 5–12.* Mountain View, CA: Mayfield.

Silva, L., Arlyn, J., & Beenen, E. (2008). What does healthy really mean? *Horace, 24*(2), 1–3.

Simovska, V. (2004). Student participation: A democratic education perspective—experience from the health promoting schools in Macedonia. *Health Education Research, 19*(2), 198–207.

Slattery, P., & Dees, D. (1998). In W. Pinar (Ed.), *The passionate mind of Maxine Greene: "I am—not yet."* (pp. 14–29). London, UK: Falmer Press.

Smith, D. (1999). *Pedagon: Interdisciplinary essays in the human sciences, pedagogy, and culture.* New York, NY: Peter Lang.

Smith, D. (2008a). *Wisdom responses to globalization: A meditation on Ku-Shan.* Presentation to Simon Fraser University, Faculty of Education, April 8, 2008.

Smith, D. (2008b). "The farthest west is but the farthest east:" The long way of Oriental/ Occidental engagement. In C. Eppert & H. Wang, *Cross-cultural studies in curriculum: Eastern thought, educational insights* (pp. 1–34). New York, NY: Taylor & Francis.

Smith, D. (2008c). Leo Strauss to collapse theory: Considering the neoconservative attack on modernity and the work of education. *Critical Studies in Education, 49*(1), 33–48.

Smith, D. (2011a). Can wisdom trump the market as a basis for education? In D. Stanley & K. Young (Eds.), *Contemporary studies in Canadian curriculum: Principles, portraits, and practices* (pp. 153–186). Calgary, AB: Detselig.

Smith, D. (2011b). *Advanced research seminar in curriculum research.* (Unpublished course syllabus). Edmonton: University of Alberta.

Smith, D. (2013). Wisdom responses to globalization. In W. Pinar (Ed.), *The International Handbook of Curriculum Research.* (2nd ed.) (pp. 45–59). New York, NY: Routledge.

Smith, S. (1992). Studying the lifeworld of physical education: A phenomenological orientation. In A. C. Sparkes (Ed.), *Research in physical education and sport: Exploring alternative visions* (pp. 61–89). London, UK: Falmer Press.

Sparkes, A. (1994). Life histories and the issue of voice: Reflections on an emerging relationship. *International Journal of Qualitative Studies in Education, 7*, 165–183.

Sparkes, A. (1995). Writing people. *Quest, 47*, 158–195.

Sparkes, A. (1999) Exploring body narratives. *Sport, Education and Society, 4*(1), 17–30.

Sparkes, A. (2002). *Telling tales in sport and physical activity: A qualitative journey.* Champaign, IL: Human Kinetics.

Sparkes, A., & Templin, T. (1992). Life histories and physical education teachers: Exploring the meanings of marginality. In A. C. Sparkes (Ed.), *Research in physical education and sport: Exploring alternative visions.* London, UK: Falmer Press.

St. Leger, L. (2004). What's the place of schools in promoting health? Are we too optimistic? *Health Promotion Journal, 19*(4), 405–408.

Stenhouse, L. (1975). *An introduction to curriculum research and development.* London, UK: Heinemann.

Storey, K., et al. (2009). Diet quality, nutrition and physical activity among adolescents: The Web-SPAN (Web-Survey of Physical Activity and Nutrition) project. *Public Health Nutrition, 12*(11), 2009–2017.

Stringer, E. (2008). *Action research in education* (2nd ed.). Upper Saddle River, NJ: Pearson.

Sumara, D., & Carson, T. (1997). *Action research as a living practice.* New York, NY: Peter Lang.

Thompson, S., & Gifford, S. (2000). Trying to keep a balance: The meaning of health and diabetes in an urban Aboriginal community. *Social Science and Medicine, 51*, 1457–1472.

Thornburn, M., Jess, M., & Atencio, M. (2011). Thinking differently about curriculum: Analyzing the potential contribution of physical education as part of "health and well-being" during a time of revised curriculum ambitions in Scotland. *Physical Education and Sport Pedagogy, 16*(4), 383–398.

Tibbetts, K., Faircloth, S., Nee-Benham, M., & Pfeiffer, T. (2000). A shared story. In M. Nee-Benham & J. Cooper (Eds.), *Indigenous education models for contemporary practice: In our Mother's voice* (Vol. II) (pp. 123–134). New York, NY: Routledge.

Tinning, R. (1997). Performance and participation discourses in human movement: Toward a socially critical physical education. In J. Fernandez-Balboa (Ed.), *Critical postmodernism in human movement, physical education, and sport.* Albany: State University of New York Press.

Tinning, R. (2004). Conclusion: Ruminations on body knowledge and control and the spaces for hope and happening. In J. Evans, B. Davies, & J. Wright (Eds.), *Body knowledge and control: Studies in the sociology of physical education and health* (pp. 218–238). London, UK: Routledge.

Tinning, R. (2010). *Pedagogy and human movement: Theory, practice, research.* London, UK: Routledge.

Tinning, R., & Glasby, T. (2002). Pedagogical work and the "cult of the body": Considering the role of HPE in the context of the "new public health." *Sport, Education & Society, 7*(2), 109–119.

Toelken, B. (1976). Seeing with a Native eye: How many sheep will it hold? In W. Capps & E. Tonsing (Eds), *Seeing with a Native eye: Essays on Native American religion* (pp. 9–24). New York, NY: Harper and Row.

Tremblay, M., Shields, M., Laviolette, M., Craig, C., Janssen, I., & Gorber, S. (2010). *Fitness of Canadian children and youth: Results from the 2007–2009 Canadian Health Measures Survey. Health Reports, 21*(1), 21–35. Retrieved from http://www.statcan.gc.ca/pub/82-003-x/2010001/article/11065-eng.pdf

U.S. Department of Agriculture. (2010). *Dietary guidelines for Americans* (7th ed.). Washington, DC: US Government Printing Office. Retrieved from http://health.gov/dietaryguidelines/dga2010/DietaryGuidelines2010.pdf

Wang, H. (2010). The temporality of *currere*, change, and teacher education. *Pedagogies: An International Journal, 5*(4), 275–285.

well. (n.d.). Online etymology dictionary. Retrieved from http://www.etymonline.com/index. php?allowed_in_frame=0&search=well&searchmode=none

Welwood, J. (1992). *Ordinary magic: Everyday life as a spiritual path.* Boston, MA: Shambhala.

Westerman, F. Red Crow. (2008). *Indigenous Native American prophecy: Elders speak, part 1.* (4:35–6:15). Retrieved from http://www.youtube.com/watch?v=g7cylfQtkDg

Whitehead, M. (1990). Meaningful existence, embodiment and physical education. *Journal of Philosophy of Education, 24*(1), 3–13.

Winter, R. (2003). Buddhism and action research: Towards an appropriate model of inquiry for the caring professions. *Educational Action Research, 11*(1), 141–155.

AUTHOR INDEX

SUBJECT INDEX

Y

Z

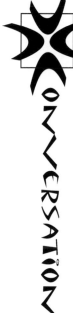

OMPLICATED

A BOOK SERIES OF CURRICULUM STUDIES

Reframing the curricular challenge educators face after a decade of school deform, the books published in Peter Lang's Complicated Conversation Series testify to the ethical demands of our time, our place, our profession. What does it mean for us to teach now, in an era structured by political polarization, economic destabilization, and the prospect of climate catastrophe? Each of the books in the Complicated Conversation Series provides provocative paths, theoretical and practical, to a very different future. In this resounding series of scholarly and pedagogical interventions into the nightmare that is the present, we hear once again the sound of silence breaking, supporting us to rearticulate our pedagogical convictions in this time of terrorism, reframing curriculum as committed to the complicated conversation that is intercultural communication, self-understanding, and global justice.

The series editor is

Dr. William F. Pinar
Department of Curriculum Studies
2125 Main Mall
Faculty of Education
University of British Columbia
Vancouver, British Columbia V6T 1Z4
CANADA

To order other books in this series, please contact our Customer Service Department:

(800) 770-LANG (within the U.S.)
(212) 647-7706 (outside the U.S.)
(212) 647-7707 FAX

Or browse online by series:

www.peterlang.com